Ninjutsu

The Ninjutsu Traditions of the Ninja

(The Ultimate Guide to the Secret History of the Ninja)

Anna Wright

Published By **Oliver Leish**

Anna Wright

All Rights Reserved

Ninjutsu: The Ninjutsu Traditions of the Ninja (The Ultimate Guide to the Secret History of the Ninja)

ISBN 978-1-77485-630-7

No part of this guidebook shall be reproduced in any form without permission in writing from the publisher except in the case of brief quotations embodied in critical articles or reviews.

Legal & Disclaimer

The information contained in this ebook is not designed to replace or take the place of any form of medicine or professional medical advice. The information in this ebook has been provided for educational & entertainment purposes only.

The information contained in this book has been compiled from sources deemed reliable, and it is accurate to the best of the Author's knowledge; however, the Author cannot guarantee its accuracy and validity and cannot be held liable for any errors or omissions. Changes are periodically made to this book. You must consult your doctor or get professional medical advice before using any of the suggested remedies, techniques, or information in this book.

Upon using the information contained in this book, you agree to hold harmless the Author from and against any damages, costs, and expenses, including any legal fees potentially resulting from the application of any of the information provided by this guide. This disclaimer applies to any damages or injury caused by the use and application, whether directly or indirectly, of any advice or information presented, whether for breach of contract, tort, negligence, personal injury, criminal intent, or under any other cause of action.

You agree to accept all risks of using the information presented inside this book. You need to consult a professional medical practitioner in order to ensure you are both able and healthy enough to participate in this program.

TABLE OF CONTENTS

Introduction

As silent as the night. As fast as a whirlwind of wind. As deadly as a concealed blade. These images immediately pop to mind when you mention of "ninja". These warriors from the past of Japanese mythology have captured the hearts and imaginations of millions of people from all over the world.

What do you need to do in order to be one of these secretive warriors in the modern world? Do you think it is possible to remain hidden from the world and deceive your adversaries?

This guide will teach you the hidden side of ninjas as well as their revered practice of the ninjutsu. This manual will teach you the different skills, techniques and the mindsets that create the professional ninja.

Self-defense, mental and emotional evocation this guide will provide you with the details that have been inaccessible to the general public for decades. From the thick forests of the ancient Japan Now, you can learn what it takes to be an Ninja.

This guide will provide information on tactics, weapons, as well as training strategies to help you begin your journey towards becoming one of the most deadly groups of warriors that the world has ever seen.

We hope that you take in this book and start your journey as Shinobi of the future!

Chapter 1: The Introduction Of Ninjutsu

Espionage, stealth and sabotage.

These are the thoughts that pop into your the mind when ninjas are mentioned in the conversation.

The legend says that they rose to power during the chaos during the Japanese Sengoku time period Ninjas have claimed deadlines that are on equal to the mastery of the Samurai. Instructed to defeat the most proud warriors and fend off death with the speed of their breathing, ninjas are the story of legends.

There is little information about the history of ninjas, and their dark practice of Ninjutsu. Some say it was started in an attempt to stay on the pace the Chinese and Korean assassins who were attempting to take down those who were in the position of power and transfer favor to certain lords.

There is also a belief that ninjutsu originated from the desire to discover an alternative to bushido and the methods of the noble warriors who were willing to sacrifice their lives for their masters.

NINJUTSU TODAY

It is widely recognized as a fighting art, the ninjutsu concentrates on securing the mind and transforming the body into an effective weapon equipped to wield short-range swords, chained blades, and chained weapons to bows and the arrow.

In addition to the skill of mastering weapons, ninjutsu focuses on kicking, grappling and the ancient form of taijutsu. It is made up of simple skills developed to deter and permanently silence enemies.

In our modern society the ninja is still a in popular culture. They are romanticized and portrayed in earlier versions; shadows that move through the night's darkness with various techniques to take down their victims.

You can find them in Japanese television dramas and cartoons. There are times when you can see the characters in Asian action films. Their appeal has not been diminished and their secret art is considered to be among the most deadly in the field.

INTRODUCING NINJUTSU

In the past there was no way to have any say in becoming an Ninja. When you came from a clan of ninjas and you were born into it, you had the chance to learn the art from your ancestors. It was impossible to choose a different job.

In the past, Ninjas had to be blacksmiths and farmers in their respective communities, however their practice and art were their main focus.

A lot of families were classified as shinobi clans, which were able to compete for the top warriors. Families would fight against each other to win the respect of their lords, and pitting their best in battles of wits and endurance.

They trained in private, away from the any scrutiny that might discover their methods and secrets. Ninjutsu was taught in the early years of early childhood, at the time the child was capable of walking, running and control weapons.

Like the samurai the discipline of intense and constant practicing and mastery were everyday goals of shinobi the training. Each moment is dedicated to perfecting of their craft , an authentic Japanese-inspired practice.

Many descendants of clans known as shinobi have opened their doors their doors to others and have shared their knowledge. There are lessons available at various martial arts institutions as part of their routine. But here, you can learn this art in the convenience of your own living room.

Ninjutsu 101: The Basic misconceptions about Ninja Training

If that was not their primary goal, they wouldn't be able to eliminate all people within a specific zone. If their goal was to pursue a specific person, they'd employ every method to avoid the detection of others until they come in the vicinity of their mark.

It would create quite trouble if they were to notify everyone in the zone of the presence, by engaging all those they encounter. This is why taijutsu became extremely important. It allowed them to pick their battles, while also keeping the track of their priorities.

Another thing that many have been unable to grasp about ninjutsu is that it's one huge school run by a single master and a group of highly skilled students. This isn't the reality.

While at one time there were many of practitioners, these Ninjas weren't unison. Certain clans were at war against each other, while others had different lords who were on opposite side of the coin.

There were around nine major Ninjutsu schools in the past times, each having their own imitators and sub-schools, which made the family tree more complicated.

Another myth about ninjutsu is that it doesn't specifically employ the techniques of sorcery and black magic. In the end, Ninjas were just ordinary Japanese people who lived in unique situations.

The rumors of disappearing and changing are just romanticized exaggerations about their capabilities intended to confuse and incite anxiety. It's surprising to discover that it was the ninjas who spread these myths about their capabilities. The less people knew about their abilities the more potent their methods were.

In this book, ninjas utilize various techniques and tools that could appear too easy to be efficient. If properly trained and disciplined this method were the norm for lethality and stealth during the ancient Japanese time.

One of the biggest misconceptions that people are prone to about ninjutsu is the idea that it teaches or demands insane amounts of speed.

Primarily, ninjutsu's focus isn't about speed. It's about being able to survive. Training isn't meant to make you a breeze over opponents and watch them fall on you. Ninjutsu training was developed to help outnumbered people who were in a hostile environment. That's why ninjas were also taught to be tolerant of pain. They would take a break on purpose and expose themselves to extreme cold and extreme heat in order to prepare themselves for the worst-case scenario.

The Ninja relied on stealth deceit, and guerilla tactics since they were the tools that could help them get through the conflicting Sengoku time. While they are viewed as unworthy and a detriment to the elite samurai, Ninja have proved that their creativity can sometimes outweigh force and skill.

It's sad that many popular depictions of ninjas have them depicted as villains and wicked Henchmen. It is likely due to their famous rivalry with Samurai, who were all about honour and justice. The truth is they were a oppressed group of people who were doing their best to endure the brutality of the history of their nation.

The 8 GATE OF NINJA

If you decide to leave aside other fundamental disciplines such as kendo or Aikido, which are included in the shinobi-training program, you'll end up with a huge body of specific training ideas and techniques. The whole collection of information is referred to as the eight gates.

Each gate represents a distinct aspect of ninjutsu that ranges from the equipment employed to the hidden mystic arts. Mastery is possible when a shinobi commits to mastering the art and passing through each gate like they are embarking on a path to mastery.

KIAI-JUTSU

The first gate is often regarded as the most important in the realm of knowledge, this one is about the use of sound and language to strengthen the body. From mantras and shouts as well as body language, and symbolic meaning Shinobis will be taught the ways to tap into their personal energy and influence the energy of their adversaries.

NINPO-TAIJUTSU

This is the part of using your body as a weapon for self-defense. It's not just about the part which requires physical exercise. It's also about the allocation of energy for specific tasks, allowing you to have enough power to take on your adversaries. Also, it involves training your mind to determine the most effective way to complete certain tasks, like climbing walls or holding a an extended breath under water. It is all about the idea of conserving energy.

NINJA NO KEN

This covers all types of mastery using the sword. Although it is thought to be similar to warriors of the samurai with their Katana, the ninja have developed a unique approach to swordsmanship. Contrary to what is commonly believed that the ninja don't employ the same weapons like the Samurai.

The samurai had larger and more curving swords due to the fact that they could access better materials, and they were only intended for use in combat. However the ninja were also able to use their swords as tools that meant they required access to more materials and a greater functions. Their blades were much longer and straighter. This made them better for the stabbing motions.

They can also sink their swords into the ground with the help of the handles to provide an initial boost to climb higher levels.

Additionally the ninjas also utilized shorter blades to make it easier to block attacks by opponents, specifically the samurai. They open up the attack and then swoop in closer to deliver their own final strike.

Ninja were not trained only to master their own swords, but also to utilize other swords to defeat their adversaries. This could include different ninjas, or even Samurai. They are specialists in both areas and are knowledgeable about the techniques used by Samurai warriors too.

SHURIKEN-JUTSU

This section is about the use by ninjas of the shuriken weapon, which is popular and well-known. The weapon is a flat disc of steel typically in the form of the shape of a star. The weapon is long ranged which is thrown at crucial places to kill or destroy an opponent. In this way, ninjas can focus and increase their speed of throwing to be in a position to throw numerous shuriken in order to cover a large space.

They also learn to use steel spikes , which could be used as tools for climbing, as to trap opponents who are about to come, and even as weapons. They learn to join spikes to their limbs in order to increase the force of their Taijutsu.

SOO-JUTSU

The ninjas' mastery of spears of all kinds; not only for combat, but also for mobility. The extended range of a spear gives them an advantage when fighting. They also have been trained to shoot spears and aim them across great distances in order to strike distant adversaries.

They are also taught to utilize them as measurement instruments to determine the depth of bodies of water or utilize as a climbing device.

KA-JUTSU

Incredibly, none other martial art combines methods of using fire in the same way as the ninjutsu. It covered learning to master fire in all forms and uses. From making use of smoke as a disguise or distraction in the creation of weapons that spit flames, ninjas are trained to use the destructive power of nature to take their own actions.

It was also believed that ninjas were able to inhale fire by spitting oil onto a torch that was lit. They've been taught to utilize the surroundings to their advantage. This included fire as well as anything else they can think of.

NINJA NO UGEI

This is possibly the most popular part of becoming the Ninja. This is the art of fooling enemies with various techniques. The popular culture makes many believing that stealth was the sole skill of the Ninja. While hiding behind camouflage or the dark night was their specialty however, this gate did more than just that.

In the real sense of espionage also learned to deceive in battle. They could trick their opponents into believe that they will follow the correct path however, they would surprise them with an elaborate plan. They were taught the art of deceit to fool others into their traps.

Ninjas were also taught manipulatives and impersonations. It is unlikely to have a skilled ninja appear to you, however the most skilled ninja may already be close to you, without realizing it.

NINJA NO KIYOMON

As the last entry point to complete mastery, this section examines the real mindset of the Ninja. The mind was the most powerful weapon, and they taught their minds to see every possible angle to gain an advantage.

For a ninja there is no limit to what they can achieve. They can build their self-confidence and confidence quickly, increasing the chances of success and their chances of survival. They approach every challenge with an open heart to discover ways to remain ahead.

These ideas are also embraced by motivational speakers to inspire individuals. It is interesting to note that a ninjutsu inspired mindset is thought to be a powerful tool to achieve success.

In this guide, you will be introduced to the different ways of thinking and practices that are represented by the eight gates. You will discover the steps to becoming Ninjas, not only through Coplay however, but through actual action too.

Chapter 2: Spirit And Kiai

It is considered to be the most basic principle of all Japanese arts of combat, the concept of kiai has been utilized by other masters of the eastern arts to build up the stamina and increase confidence.

In the base, every warrior is blessed with an inner strength that they use when they are engaged. The power of this spirit is a reflection of the power of their determination to defeat their foes. The less strong the spirit and the less determination to fight.

It is the art Kiai is about strengthening the spirit by shouting. It may seem simple and absurd initially, but the truth is that true masters could be able to talk for hours about how crucial it is to strengthen the spirit prior to studying any training techniques or techniques.

If you translate kiai in English the meaning changes to "the connection in energy". This is the essence that this practice is. It is about creating energy and channeling it into fight.

THE HORSE SQUAT

When you are a beginner ninja you need to build your passion for winning as warrior. It is about approaching battles with the aim of walking through the other side with victory. In order to help you get yourself in a positive mindset Kiai can be employed to boost your self-confidence.

The best part to note is there's no single way to build your personal Kiai. Every person has their own spirit, therefore, there are many methods to develop a unique spirit.

For a kiai practice to improve your kiai, you must be in the squat horse position. Different forms of marital arts from the east view this posture as the fundamental principle of all forms of training.

Place your feet in a half-squatting posture. This will place your legs and feet in a squat. Make sure that both feet are on the ground. With your legs separated and straight back, keep your legs in a straight line by bending your arms and keeping them to your sides.

Before you do any other workout, it is crucial to be in this position in order to activate Kiai. This will help you strengthen yourself and boost confidence.

BREATHING

It's not just a shout. It's a method of attracting energy and establishing it within your own. Begin by taking a few slow breaths. Be aware of you taking energy from the surroundings. Allow the breath to enter your body and increase the oxygen levels in your muscles.

After a few breaths, you can use your Kiai. It isn't necessary to shout out a specific phrase or word. A single, strong syllable will suffice. For those who are new to the game, start by saying "HA!"

PROPER EXECUTION

In contrast to other types that shout, can't shout out of your throat. You draw it from your diaphragm.

It's also advisable to maintain a straight neck to create a clear pathway to breathe. Take a deep breath through the nose , and feel the energy rise in your.

When you yell "HA!" paint a mental picture that bolsters your resolve. It could be a photo that shows you breaking through a block or kicking an attacker. It could be also an image of your muscles getting stronger. It must be a picture that gives you confidence in you.

What you want to hear is a clear kiai which can be heard throughout the room. A shout for battle is intended to "psyche" yourself to face the battle. Do not be concerned if the message does not come off as powerful as you wanted it to be.

For those who are new to the sport learning this form, it requires some time and effort. The more you practice, the bigger your lungs will get and the greater bass you get from your Kiai.

The hallmark of a great kiai lies in its impact on adversaries. It sounds intimidating and frightening. It shows them that you're committed to winning and that you're prepared for any eventuality.

Watch some professional and masters demonstrate their Kiai on Youtube. You will notice that they are more powerful and solid when they call out their Kiai. The reason for this is that the aim for the battle cry is focus the focus of your mind and supply you with confidence.

Note that reciting your kiai's name is not intended to provoke anger. It's intended to inspire you to be more determined. Your movements and your blows get more deliberate and your intention becomes clear through your actions.

At higher levels, you'll also often invoke your kiai whenever you are striking, kicking, and connecting blows to an opponent. There's a huge debate over whether using kiai to attack will make your attack more powerful. It is not necessary to be concerned about this as long as you invoke the affect on you.

Chapter 3: Beginner Ninja Concepts And Weapons

Shinobi were not feared due to their timeframes, some of the first techniques taught to them focus on shifting across battles. They were trained to focus on the art of evasion and escape from battle and were able to focus their tasks without creating much of a fuss.

Taijutsu is where it is useful. The art is using your body as a weapon of self-defense. In combination with tricks and other techniques Taijutsu is thought of to be one of the most surprising methods to win or leave your adversaries confused and in awe of where you are.

One of the biggest misconceptions about Ninjas was that they are made to kill machines that could not distinguish between enemy and target. In reality they were among the most intelligent fighters of the past of Japan.

Ninja Levels

The training hierarchy of their employees reflected their rational approach. The lowest level is Genin. Genin are students who are near-completers of their basic education however they are required to perform certain tasks.

Due to their inexperience and lack of training, they are typically assigned safer tasks like reconnaissance and information gathering. They can observe their targets from a distance, and submit brief reports for their masters or lords, who decide to assign the next mission to a more skilled Shinobi.

After a Genin has demonstrated the potential and dedication to training and their job then they can move to Chonin. At this level they are assigned more dangerous assignments, where they target targets in more secure areas. They are also chosen as aids to more advanced Ninjas to take on more risky assignments.

In the end finally, a Chonin changes into an Jonin after they've achieved enough points and their master decides it's time to confer the title. Jonin can perform everything from sabotage, espionage, and sabotage reconnaissance. They are able to conduct their own research, planning and even execute provided they've been granted the authority by their Lord.

Shinobi typically get the most hazardous assignments, including assassinations or murders of famous people or infiltrations into enemy camps. Their abilities are highly valued and are seen as valuable assets to any Lord. They are regarded as highly favored by the ninjas, particularly in cases where they've contributed a lot to their country. They also bring honour to their clan of shinobi when their Jonin are able to win the approval of their Lord.

Ninja Weapons

One of the factors that distinguished the ninja from other martial artists at the time was the kind of tools and weapons they used. While the ninja used bows and swords, just as samurai however, they also had other tools that gave them an advantage over their opponents in battle.

The Shuko

Infrequently seen in artists' drawings the shuko consisted of a thin sheet of metal that was worn on the knuckles. As this cured the palm's back along with the palm. Spikes were placed on the palm for two reasons.

One was that it made climbing difficult surfaces much easier, as the spikes offered a form of traction on these surfaces. Ninjas could cling to walls for short amounts of time, which gave them an advantage in height over their competitors.

Second, the spikes as well as sheet of metal served as excellent weapons at close range. Ninjas had the ability to leave deep scratches on their adversaries or break jaws with the shuko.

The Shuriken

The one that is most well-known to both practitioners and enthusiasts. The discs with a star shape were simple to create and let ninjas make the most of the tiny amount of steel that came their way.

If they were directed to the right areas, ninjas may be able to take down unarmed adversaries. When on the battlefield however, helmets made head strikes virtually impossible using the shuriken. That's why ninjas favored these discs for their maiming capabilities that were aimed at joints and limbs in order to defeat the larger and more heavily-armed opponents.

The Caltrops Caltrops

They were thought of as cleverly designed spike traps, which are very simple to set up. Made up of a single metal point that had four spikes protruding from it Ninjas employed the tools to construct traps to stop pursuers who are on the trail.

The concept behind the tools was designed to ensure that, when they're dropped, they will always land on a sharp spike that is pointed upwards. The Ninja could just throw several caltrops onto an area and they would all cause injury to anyone who was stepping upon them.

The weight and Chain

It was thought to be among the weapon types developed by the ninjas it was made up of a long chain that turned for a long distance. At one end of the chain was a heavy metal object that was fixed to the link that was the last within the chain.

When an ninja, they would throw the end of the chain that was weighted chain at their targets to snag their weapons or knock them down. If an opponent blocks the chain using their arm or sword and the chain wraps around the weapon or arm because of the change in direction that occurs on the weight, which causes the weapon to gain grip against the adversary.

In this scenario in this position, a strong pull is enough to disarm or push the adversary towards the ninja and knock them off balance. This is the reason this weapon was popular among Ninjas when fighting the techniques of the Samurai.

The Kusarigama

This is a better version of the chain and weight that came with a tiny sickle at the opposite part of the chain. Similar principles apply in this case; the chain is used to draw opponents closer by using the edge of the chain that is weighted.

With the sickle at the other hand the ninja may deliver an unfathomable blow and cut the appendage off of an adversary after they've drawn their attention to the Ninja. The ninjas no longer needed to change weapons as they was already a sword in their backs in the form of the sickle.

While it was convenient however, it was difficult to use due to the fragile nature of the chain. It took many years of instruction to be able to use the weapon efficiently.

The Kunai

This is now described as the "utility knife" of the Ninja. The dagger was an ninja-like tool with a small holes of metal at the other side of the handle.

This weapon was created for close-range as well as projectile combat. It could be thrown as darts or used as daggers for shooting. They could also be employed to climb fences or as wedges to serve other purposes.

The Tekko-Kagi

Like the Shuko similar to the Shuko, this was a set of spikes affixed to a bar of metal to allow the ninja to grip. This was originally an instrument for farmers to get rid of the weeds that grew on his property.

Ninjas wore the weapons at both sides. Their fists would become powerful weapons that could snare the blade that was incoming and scratch off enemy faces with just a single swipe.

They were also employed to decimate opponents. When a blow is resisted the ninja would then plunge the left claw to the body their opponent, and then follow it up with the right. Once both claws are engaged and the ninja is ready to tear their opponent in pieces, similar to opening a cabinet.

The Nekode

The term "nekode" originated from the word neko, meaning cat. They were iron thimbles designed to fit each finger. Each thimble features a small spike on its end.

If put on the fingers the ninja may utilize the nekode to scratch at their foes. They typically coat these thimbles with poison in order to enhance the power that the weapon has.

The main difference between the other claws lies in the fact they were simple to hide. Instead of carrying heavy claws, people would often prefer to carry thimbles since they were simpler to carry and use. They were the weapon that were used for infiltrations and assassinations.

Shikoro. Shikoro

As a key to unlocking a ninja's locks the small saw with two edges aids ninjas in navigating through doors that were barred by wooden planks. After a rigorous education, the Ninja could cut through gates and fences easily, granting the ability to access their targets.

One of the things about this piece is that it was not constructed as an actual saw, but more like a dagger with sharp edges. This means that it was as a tool rather as opposed to a weapon. However, it could also be shot from a distance towards an unattainable target.

The Blowgun

In all types of guerilla warfare, guns were also a popular choice for the ninjas. Because it was possible for a ninja to use the weapon from a safe distance and instantly take down an enemy or guard without alarming.

The blowguns used by the Japanese were typically bamboo shoots. Bamboo was their preferred material since the plant was already hollow in the beginning. It was an issue of smoothing the edges to ensure that people could put it into their mouths.

To shoot shots, the ninja utilized needles or spikes of a large size which were coated with poison. With the right aim the ninja was able to take out an opponent from a distance of several yards without the opponent being aware of the Ninja. This weapon let them remain hidden in the shadows, and remain undetected.

NINJAS AND FIRE

Incredibly, ninjas were not novices to the power of fire on the battlefield. If their cover was destroyed or they were required to destroy a structure or a crowd of persons, they would not spend their energy on weapons that required them to take on people one at one at a at a. They often used fire to cause destruction over vast areas, and then spread fear on the surrounding people.

This is the reason why Ninja always had tools with them that they could make fire. There was a saying that regardless of the type of job they performed they would always have the fire source on them, for example, the hidane.

It was a tiny wooden pipe, which contained a tiny burning wire and an extremely potent fuel. The ninja could immediately ignite objects without going through the hassle of creating an ignition.

This might be the prehistoric Japanese equivalent to today's lighter. Although cigarettes were not widely used in Japan in the past however, there were plenty of ways to start small fires.

Apart from their hidane, Ninja were also aware of the potential of certain materials to catch on fire. This is why they'd carry around flint stones as well as other spark sources which to ignite in the event that they did not have hidane with them.

With the aid of fire Ninjas can set the arrows' ends into flames and set buildings in flames from far away. They can start flames in castle gardens, and create a distraction for guards. They can also throw burning fuel at their enemies, setting people on to catch fire.

NINJAS AND POISIONS

Although they are considered to be weak in the martial arts The ninja did not hesitate to use the force of nature to defeat their foes in the dark of night.

It is also part of the legends that put Ninjas on a completely different level of ingenuity when compared with the blacksmiths and samurai from the Sengoku period. This is due to the fact that on the top of martial arts and guns, the warriors were educated on poisons and cures.

Utilizing various seeds of fruit Ninjas were able to get rid of cyanide by pressing them and drying them, based on their understanding about the fruits. They also knew that certain leaves of plants contained poisons , such as tomatoes leaves and the rhubarb. The farmers would grow these vegetables and harvest them for their fruit and poison.

In some cases, the ninjas would also receive their poisons from animals who produced their own poison to defend themselves. This meant they were aware of poisonous scorpions, spiders, snakes, and even Frogs. They would capture the animals, breed them, and take their poisons on a regularly. Ninjas always had an abundance of poisons to choose from.

One specific poison that was specific to the Japanese was the blowfish poison. The fish is considered to be one of the most rare and dangerous foods in Japan. Chefs were required to go through specific training to prepare the fish in so that diners were able to enjoy the unique flavor of the poison without being afflicted by its toxicity.

Ninjas were adept at taking this poison from fish, and were popular for assassination. This is due to the fact that this poison isn't as difficult to extract as cyanide which was a tiny amount from seeds of fruits. There was a lot of puffer fish found in many areas of water as fishermen would throw them back into the sea whenever they could take one in. In addition blowfish poison is extremely powerful, capable of killing individuals in the tiniest of doses.

With poison as their weapon the ninjas used poison to use them in various ways. One strategy was to get into the kitchen of a castle where food was being cooked. When the cooks weren't watching at the kitchen, a ninja might introduce toxic ingredients into food being cooked. They could then infect large numbers of people without needing to raise their knives against anyone.

Another option was to coat their weapons with poison. Everything that was sharp for a ninja was likely to be coated with some type of poison. From their swords, to their darts, even their claws.

In addition, ninjas would pour intoxicants directly onto the lips of their sleep victims at late at night. As they hung from the ceiling, they would spray their poisons onto the string, which would then hang over the mouths of their sleeping targets.

Chapter 4: The Art Of Stealth

Don't worry about smoke bombs or intricate wallpapers. Nowadays, the concept that stealth is a concept has evolved dramatically. In ancient Japanese time, ninjas had darkness in which they could blend in, making it easier for them to infiltrate houses and castles undetected to commit their targets.

However, the art of concealment isn't just about having black clothes and waiting for the night to fall. Actually, it's among the more intriguing ways to train as Shinobi. The school of stealth is centered around manipulating and analyzing your position against the presence of other people and allowing you to walk around without provoking suspicion.

THE BASICS

How Can Others Identify You

A key thing you'll be able to comprehend about stealth is the best way to disguise your identity, but rather how easy it is to expose yourself to others. Knowing how your adversaries will notice your presence is just half the battle that you have won already.

Naturally, we can recognize the presence of things by their senses. The most frequently used resources are the eyes, ears , and the nose. The initial part of stealth training is tricking your senses to make others believe that you're not in the room.

The Eyes Play with the Eyes

To be able to see the eyes, it is necessary to keep in mind three aspects that can make someone pay attention to you:

Silhouettes

Movements

Colors

In addition to blinding your adversaries by bright smoke or light Ninjas also make use of darkness to help them move. The three elements into a single base; black. It's difficult to distinguish the silhouettes of a person and to detect motion in a dark setting. It's also difficult to discern colours apart when you're wearing black clothing in dark areas.

Additionally, ninjas practice some specific practices to help them plan their movement plan during a task.

They first know the source of light. The first thing that a ninja will do during reconnaissance is to discover the areas where light is present in a specific region. This allows them to plan the best places to go and not to be.

The next thing they take note of is where they can see people. Being around other people can pose the possibility of a threat to their privacy. They don't want to be seen unless they are forced to do so by option.

For a ninja, there's always a way which leads to their goal without risk of being spotted. This led to the romantic picture of ninjas scaling walls and soaring over rooftops, where there is no artificial light and no other people. Their minds are taught to shift perspectives instantly which allows them to discover unusual solutions to common problems.

They then move slower. They know that speed can cause them to miss important things or make unplanned movements. Don't think about the image of ninjas who move at a dazzling speed to confuse their adversaries. They move slow to avoid creating an impression of motion, which can raise suspicion.

The Ears and Playing

As a result of their slow pace and slowed down, the ninja also took advantage of the sounds that were prevalent in the surroundings in order to benefit from the surroundings. It was common to take small animals during missions, including kittens and dogs which could be used as effective distractions.

When the animals move around and are detected they take advantage of the opportunity to quickly move and gain more ground. Ninjas also make use of background sounds like the sound of streams of water or the crackling of leaves at night to disguise the sound that they make from their steps.

When walking on unsteady areas, they employ cloths to cover the surface to reduce the sound that their footsteps could produce.

They're so aware of their actions that their shoes were different from those of the typical Japanese warrior. They had thicker padding, and lesser covering on their sandals in order to make the minimum amount of noise while they walked. Contrary to the samurai, who were loud and wore vibrant colors, the ninjas ensured that everything they did worked perfectly with their purpose.

MODERN DAY Stealth

In our modern-day urban society lights are everywhere and you can be able to see you from miles away. Donning a ninja costume will only make a shinobi standout even more.

This is where costumes and impersonation are in. The dark does not have to be the principal stage for the ninja, that they blend into effortlessly. They now appear like normal people walking through the crowds. They're still capable of being hidden from view.

They are able to do this since they perceive environments as having a myriad of elements they can utilize to advantage. They can use challenges as an opportunity for them to test innovative strategies to confuse their adversaries.

Misdirection and distraction are important players in the present. Have you noticed the manner in which street magicians perform? They're able to hold your attention to a particular spot, even in an extremely busy street. As a modern shinobi you could also use distraction techniques to draw people's attention to something else while you walk along. It's all about the way you view a particular scenario.

Chapter 5: The Art Of Subterfuge

Most often viewed as a negative behavior today, subterfuge played a significant influence on the development of Japanese society throughout the Sengoku period.

Alongside the stealth aspect, subterfuge was a important aspect of shinobi training. Alongside a strategy of approaching your adversaries invisibly as well as learning to trick and deceive your adversaries.

Subterfuge is a word that is a plethora of snarky synonyms like deceit or fraud. What people aren't aware of is that subterfuge also associated with shrewdness. It is the ability to leverage all the elements of your environment to your advantage, even by utilizing your adversaries themselves.

The Tenet Basic to Ninjutsu Subterfuge

A crucial task often assigned Shinobi with was reconnaissance. The gathering of information was among their specialties due to their experience in stealth. They could gather measurements and head counts, arms counts, and even the routes to attack and escape, without being noticed by enemies.

Their success did not only depend on their sleight of hand however, it was more based on their deception-related skills.

The most important thing Ninjas learn doesn't come from the dojo. They learned it on the field during missions. This lesson was taught to soldiers during battles. The the Sun Tzu's Art of War, one of the most important instructions is to learn about your opponent. That's half the battle that you win.

Ninjas could spend endless hours looking at their movements and trying to master their movements. Their mission began with their learning. Once they know everything they need to know they get to work making use of the knowledge for their benefit.

They aren't content with just the way their marks appear or what clothing they choose to wear. In addition, they take note of the lifestyles of their targets.

According to the ninja mythology the success of a task depends more on the understanding of your enemies' behavior rather than your own capabilities and tools. That meant that learning about your adversaries prior to anything else.

Invisible to many, habits can be damaging or beneficial, depending on the type of habit you've got. Once a ninja has become aware of the ways they make their target, they're well as dead.

This is due to the fact that habits are extremely difficult to challenge. They're automatic responses that your body produces without thinking. They're as natural as breathing. Ninjas make use of this to their advantage, creating targets that react with predictable patterns, taking them exactly where they'd like them to be.

Does the target's target move to left or to the right? Which foot will the mark take first to move forward when the sword is drawn? Are they confrontational or cautious? Is the mark right or left handed? What do the targets look at when in danger? Do they respond with an action of flight or fight?

These are just a few of the many aspects Shinobi will need to know while observing their targets. With this information in their fingertips, subterfuge is a breeze is a breeze.

Three Subterfuge Areas

In their training, shinobi were subjected to three different dimensions of deceit during combat. Based on the tasks assigned their way, each of the dimensions played a crucial role.

Toiri No Jutsu

This is the first of three dimensions. In this dimension, shinobi learn about how to get into areas. It could be houses, military camps castles, castles or even vehicles. Ninjas were taught a variety of strategies to gain access without alarming as they walked towards their intended targets.

One method that was popularly taught in this school was to use an alternate persona for access. As part of their routine, ninjas could often pretend to be an Buddhist monk searching for sanctuary in the temple located near the castle. In order to gain the trust of monks, over time, with written kindness, they would request to be seated with the Lord of the caste. During this time, they alter their appearance and leave their target.

Another strategy in this school was to employ females and their natural charm. In spite of the prestige and honor of being Samurai, these warriors were men by nature and could be enticed by attracted by a gorgeous woman. Ninjas used the services of women to gain details, objects, and even to get the cooperation of corrupt officials and warriors.

Chikairi No Jutsu

This area deals with sabotage during combat. In this area, ninjas were taught how to penetrate enemy camps to cause havoc and destruction on the enemy line.

Ninjas slyly break into fortresses and enemy camps in an attempt to use diverse sabotage strategies intended to destroy morale of the enemy and their survival. Certain of these actions were direct like burning down supply camps or assaulting supply vehicles. Others were indirect, like disseminating false information to the enemy line and

To gain entry Ninja were required to dress as officials, soldiers or relatives of officials, or any other person who could allow them access to enemies' lines. They also established sub-camps where they could rest and wait for their enemies to go to sleep.

After that it, it took only a few seconds to start executing their plans. It was an arson attack or a mishap, ninjas could execute their plan effortlessly, without drawing suspicion from their adversaries.

Ongyo Jutsu

After the fundamentals of destruction and entry which were discussed in the previous two dimensions, the third dimension is about ensuring an escape for the ninjas; and more importantly, their escape of themselves from intrusion.

The dimension was further subdivided into two sub-categories. One group of techniques is designed for escape strategies while the other set is intended to conceal from view.

Due to the chaos and confusion caused by their actions escape is a breeze for a ninja who has been trained. However, there are occasions in which the cover is destroyed and soldiers and government officials are aware of the plans.

If the chaos and confusion do not allow for getting away, the criminals turn on other methods to escape. This is when a small combination of stealthy skills comes to the rescue.

In black, and remaining in a tense manner The ninja may appear like trees in a large garden. They could also disguise themselves as statues for prolonged durations.

In even more hilarious situations, ninjas also have been seen taking unimaginable actions when it comes to disappearing. They have been known to conceal themselves and their family members in manure-filled jars to avoid being noticed as they concealed. Some hid behind the animals of their farms and their stalls in order they could smell the the noise of the animals could mask their breathing.

In reality the ninjas were taught to give up their pride and to sacrifice their temporary hygiene for the purpose of survival.

Basic Subterfuge Techniques

Utilizing the senses of their adversaries they are capable of sending their adversaries to other spots to take them down or draw them away from a location.

In certain situations the ninjas will throw torches or other loud items away from the location to the vicinity of an ambush or trap. Security personnel and other individuals who hear the noise would head toward the source, directing towards the area of the shinobi. This allows them to move about freely throughout the exchange.

It's also not in the nature of an shinobi's command to strike from behind. This is the largest blind spot that is a perfect to hit. Ninjas are capable of taking out any enemy and not alter them of their appearance is the best level of stealth. This allows them to go on in the dark and not let their adversaries know any more.

Ninjas also designed their own footwear that wore designs of animal paws instead of human. This was particularly helpful during instances when they were chased by a group of people. The prints of the animal would trick people into thinking those tracks weren't made by humans, which would force the shinobi to turn their attention elsewhere while the shinobi flees for safety.

It wasn't just on the battlefield that ninjas controlled using subterfuge. The clans of their clans also were well-known for inciting conflict and savagery through manipulative tactics. The heads of clans of ninjas were known to impersonate lords or politicians or force them to perform their will. Ninjas were ninjas too. the court of the Emperor was a location for deceit and sabotage.

The Secret to Subterfuge

Similar to covert operations, subterfuge can be used by creating a negative impact on your adversaries and not letting them know that you're there.

This involves completing the task in search of an advantage over others. This can only be accomplished by preparing yourself and knowing the right information. This is the reason why learning to recognize one's mark is one of the first things that a Shinobi must master.

From there they are able to manipulate or blackmail their adversaries into trusting their abilities or performing an act that the ninjas anticipate.

The essence of subterfuge is just being aware of your adversaries well enough to leverage their weaknesses against them. You capitalize on the weaknesses of your opponent and minimize their strengths. The fight is won the context of tactics rather than the sheer power. A successful victory for a ninja warrior is one where the adversary didn't know that they were on their way.

Chapter 6: The Spirituality Of The Shinobi

In popular culture, we may consider shinobi to be insanity-free, disciplined killing machines that fade into dark at the direction of their master. This is just one aspect of the Ninja. Many people are unaware that they are involved in one of the greatest struggle with their spirituality when compared to other types that are martial.

In the beginning they believed in the possibility of becoming an all-round warrior. This doesn't just apply to the warrior who has learned the required skills and techniques needed to become a ninja, but it also applies to the mental preparation and training.

This includes overcoming their own fears as well as accepting their mistakes and letting go of past mistakes , and recognizing the purpose of being a the ninja. In their personal lives they believe in forming and practicing for in order to create their own personal code of conduct called bushido.

Despite the popularity of popular culture and its myths that ninjas are also people who have goals and ideals in their lives. Although they were taught the martial art of ninjutsu from the age of just a few years and still aspiring to find a more profound feeling of purpose. This is the place where their spirituality is.

Due to their extensive background in martial arts and their determination to succeed is connected to physical and training development. They believe that with learning and continual adjustments and challenges, they'll become fully-fit warriors who are capable of overcoming any mental and physical difficulty.

The Four Gates of Spirituality

Beyond the gates to training that are the ninja's techniques and knowledge they also believe that they must traverse four mental pathways in order to free their minds from the world of ideas and unlock the true warrior in their minds.

The ninjas of the past believed that the four gates symbolized certain difficulties they would have to overcome throughout their lives. Once overcome, these gates allow new paths of thought and new perspectives on life , which would prepare them for the next challenge and the ultimate revelation.

It is interesting to note that these gates were named for the elements. They include the water, fire and earth gates as well as air and earth gates. Each gate is a specific moment during the lifetime of the Ninja. they encounter stereotyped obstacles and revelations. Each gate is marked by specific discoveries that a ninja needs to achieve by themselves without the assistance of master.

Shinobi could be stuck for many years in one place and not discover the core truths needed to progress. There are those who can get through their obstacles However, for the ninjas it was not an athletic competition. The experience was a fervent search for their authentic personas and gaining satisfaction in their work.

KUJI-IN

Apart from being a believer in the total soldier, the warriors of the ninja employed mystic art to enhance their performance in combat. The ninja believed in the mythology of hand movements that stimulated certain powers in our bodies. This art was called known as kuji-in.

In addition to boosting their strength, the ninjas also believed that the proper execution of these techniques helped to increase their senses, allowing them to see more clearly in darkness.

The essence of the kuji-in system revolves around drawing symbols by using the different locations of the fingers that also represent specific forms of energy which the ninjas could draw. The thumb was believed to be the main source of inner power and the four other fingers were the representation of the four primary elements: air, earth water, fire and earth.

For the beginner there were nine fundamental hand combinations with distinct effects on the ninja. They are as the following:

Rin provides increased resistance and strength on the body and muscles of users.

Hei was a way for ninjas hide their existence within the mind of their adversaries by preventing them from being able to recognize their own silhouettes in the darkness.

Toh brought an inner calm to ninjas particularly during times of extreme tension and pain The ninja used this symbol to keep their spirits in check.

Kai - allowed the ninja to control a large portion of their bodily functions in their mind, like heartbeat susceptibility to pain, as well as extreme temperature. They invoked this when they are they were captured and about to be beaten.

Jin - invokes the ability to telepathize that allow the ninja discern the thoughts of their adversaries and plans.

Zai creates unity with the surrounding environment and the universe. It was a common preparation routine for ninjas prior to when they embarked on risky missions.

Retsu - granted inhuman power to the ninjas, allowing them to incapacitate their adversaries by a few licks or swipes on their weapons.

Sha - This was used to stimulate the process of healing in Ninjas. If injured, and hiding the ninja invoked this pattern to help recover and return to roads at a much faster speed.

Zen - it was a different form of meditation. It offered enlightenment and greater understanding of the challenges faced by an Ninja. If they had to plan an assignment, they will use this method to assist them in determining the most effective strategy.

Alongside these nine basic patterns, this art form is made up of an array of 81 finger and hand patterns, each having their particular purpose and function.

In conjunction with their rigorous discipline and spirituality the ninjas turned out to be an extremely powerful force that caused fear in the hearts of their adversaries. In actual fact, they were very effective in their day that feudal lords were able to employ the services of ninjas at night, on top of their regular guards.

Chapter 7: The Mindset Of A Ninja

Apart from the intense physical instruction that shinobi received from their instructors They also had intensive spiritual and mental training to build their strength to fight the forces.

Although some weren't hard-core, they were as cruel. A shinobi who was who was in training would be required to gaze at the burning candle's wick for hours and hours until they would begin to experience the illusion of that they were in the flame.

They were also exposed to pain and hunger for long times to build their tolerance for discomfort. Through these experiences and trials, not only were warriors of the ninja more durable than other warriors, they developed specific mental habits which gave them an immediate advantage over the other warriors on a battlefield.

They know their limits

Nearly every ninja knows that there are occasions that they can't defeat an opponent on their own. They may be too big or fast, or even too powerful. If this happens, they'll are wise to avoid their reputations being damaged.

They take on the opponent when they appear too strong to fight on their own. They know that their objectives will be more significant than the pride they have as warriors that is why they are more willing to unite against common foes.

It's not only a matter of fights. It is also possible to climb certain heights that they can't achieve on their own. They may require an extra push or a helping helper from another Ninja. They're not afraid to join teams to accomplish their tasks.

They can alter the way they think

Due to their training in the mind Ninjas are skilled at solving the most complicated issues with ease. This isn't because they are born smart or have specialized education. They knew how to shift perceptions.

Ninjas are ninjas, and there is no limit to what they can accomplish. When they recognize an obligation that must be fulfilled, they set off to work on ways to accomplish it. If they find that their plans aren't achieving the task They don't get angry; they gain new perspectives.

For the ninjas failing is only a sign of the possibility of having other options. If the method they're using doesn't work, it indicates that they have something they've not tried yet. It is possible to quickly put aside their anger and view the problem in a different way in search of an alternative solution to the problem. They recognize the fact that their present way of thinking isn't enough to tackle a problem they require a higher quality of mind.

They appreciate the flexibility

The most viewed images of the ninjas is that they utilize bamboo shoots for breathing in the water as they wait for their prey to come through as well as for those they are following not to lose their track.

This shows their ability to adapt to the circumstances and do whatever is needed to remain on the right track. They could be in squalid areas without water or food for a long time in order to do necessary to achieve their goals.

They immediately analyze their surroundings and adapt according to their situation. In addition they don't do it right. They perform it with grace as if they've planned for such a scenario.

Legendary martial musician Bruce Lee talked about the importance of "being like water". Even though Bruce Lee wasn't a ninja the quote speaks to the importance of being flexible. Refusing to accept your current circumstances will only create more difficulties for you. If you'd like to breeze through an obstacle that is difficult then you must be in a position to ease it and erode your obstacles until they're smooth over which you can walk.

They accept pain

It's something that most people can't do due to living in a sheltered environment and the immediate pleasure. In the early days of Japan there were no modern amenities such as internet access , restaurants and spas weren't readily available. The harshness of the elements as well as the ongoing political battles that accompanied the conflicting Sengoku period.

At that time when ninjas were required to endure a rigorous and demanding training, and even more difficult missions in order to fulfill their political goals. They were not able to afford the luxury of leisure or extravagant lifestyles because they understood the importance of serving their masters.

It's not just about Ninjas, almost all martial arts have a rule or two about embracing suffering and pain on the road to success. It's not a nihilistic negative. It's a requirement for the success of a person; and ninjas taught to suffer and be miserable. This is the reason why their art form has endured through time.

They have a creative and resourceful mind.

From using bamboo leaves as breathers , to using tinder and cloth to light the fire, ninjas are been known to do a lot in a short amount of.

Because of their radical method of thinking, everyday objects are transformed into powerful weapons and tools that catch their enemies off guard. An excellent illustration is their climbing device.

Instead of making hooks from steel, which was difficult to create Ninjas used common tools for farmers like small sickles and ropes to make their hooks. Then, they utilized these hooks to climb castle walls as well as other structures.

The ninja who made popular the idea of throwing discs that were made of shurikens. With a tiny amount of steel, they could create sharp projectiles which they used to locate marks at an extended distance.

For a ninja there's nothing that is ordinary or insignificant. If they can't find a value in something, it simply means they didn't think in a way to make it work.

They were scientists who learned to learn.

It is perhaps the least known aspect of being a ninja , due to contemporary pictures that artists have created of these infamous assassins. What many people don't realize is that they are among of the most knowledgeable individuals at the time.

Ninjas were not just educated in the art of martial art, stealth, and sabotage. They also received information from the scientific community on various subjects to help them gain an advantage over their opponents.

One example is weather. Ninjas can tell they were going to have a wet night based on the appearance of clouds in earlier hours. They are able to utilize these elements to take out their foes flat-footed and soaked because of this. They are able to anticipate the requirements of their mission well before the mission begins which makes them more well-prepared as anyone else.

Another instance is their training in chemical chemistry. They were taught different combinations of materials and the results they produced. Ninjas were able to create fire from nearly anything in their immediate environment.

They could also make smoking bombs and traps and poisoned darts and arrows as well as even simple balms for bruises and wounds. They could be the whole package.

They felt incredibly confident

This was among their greatest strengths. Note that ninjas were the descendents of clandestine families who shied away from the normal world. They lived on the suburbs of towns and deep in the forests to practice their hidden skills.

The concept of honor and ego was little to a fully functioning Ninja. All they cared about was the task they intended to accomplish. They could engage a fully-armed samurai with not even a tinge of worry within their minds.

They can also smuggle into castles with full security in the event that their lord wanted them to. They have confidence in their education and abilities. They were confident that they were competent enough experience to complete the task. This is the reason they were capable of breaking down hierarchies and destabilizing systems throughout the Sengoku time period.

They were students of other Cultures

It's widely known that Japan prospered in the period when they shut off trading routes for the entire world. They remained strong and developed a steady economy in the present.

However, in the early days, Japan wasn't well-kept secret across the globe. In the provinces, a lot of previous Chinese or Korean officials would seek a ways to avoid oppression and sedition from the regime which controlled their territory.

In these regions, the customs of beliefs, concepts, beliefs and even martial arts from different countries were mingled with Japanese practices, giving birth to new ideas and methods that are very significant aspects of ninjutsu.

For the ninjas There is no difference in racial or ethnicity. The only information that was relevant was as well as irrelevant information. It didn't matter which source the idea or skill originated, so it could be applied the idea to personal situation.

Chapter 8: The Kurai Kotori Tradition

It is believed that the Kurai Kotori tradition is a way to keep very real-life abilities that are relevant to the modern world, while remaining solid to the traditions of our Japanese predecessors. The warriors who fought in the shadows of times past were aware that the secret to a successful technique was located in the application of unconventional strategies. This may be the most crucial lesson one can acquire on their way to enlightenment in combat.

FAMILY CREST

The Kurai Kotori crest takes the shape of a crow that has its wings spread across the night sky. The bird is a symbol of the warrior who is suspended above the sky and out of those of foes and secluded behind a veil of darkness and ready to strike whenever it is needed. It is the Kanji characters "Nin," which is located in the moon, is translated to mean "Sword across the chest" and the meaning of it is extremely specific.

Kurai Kotori Crest

It states that the warrior must be strong in times of difficulty and must react with determination and courage when faced with danger.

KURAI KOTORI CLAN HIERARCHY

It is crucial to be aware of the structure established in the clan. The internal workings of the Kurai Kotori clan need to be regulated if they wish functioning properly. That's why it's essential for every family member to be completely aware of the manners (reishiki) which is followed by the members. Being aware of the roles held by the clan in the clan crucial in order to comprehend the importance of organizational structure.

JONIN

The clan's leader is called the JONIN. The Jonin is the Ninja who's Ninjutsu mastery together with his leadership abilities have been dedicated to the preservation of their Kurai Kotori heritage by passing their knowledge onto new generations. Jonin Jonin is a veteran Ninja who is more than an expert of the techniques used by the clan but also moves to seek out deeper understanding of all things. The Jonin's wisdom is the one that steers the clan towards every aspect of its mission.

Jonin

JIKI DESHI

On the Jonin's side are those who have repressed their self to become a direct follower of JIKI DESHI in his principles. The Jiki Deshi's primary purpose in existence is to help their master in every way. The service allows them to gain access to exclusive information directly straight from their source. The Jiki Deshi strive to honour this clan, by being heirs to their master's name and carrying on the tradition after Jonin's death or disappearance.

Jiki Deshi

While this is a tempting path to take because of its obvious advantages however, it is that is rife with hardship. Only the most fervent warriors can endure this route for the duration of.

CHUNIN

Directly under Jonin and his selected disciples is the subordinates of his clan. They are believed to as the retainers of the clan, as well as practitioners who are highly skilled who become leaders on their own. Sub-commanders act as instructors for the people below their ranks, while also serving as a fighting force of elite when needed for a specific task.

Chunin Sub-Commanders

The sub-commander is a particular type of warrior that is accountable for the newcomers in the clan. The sub-commander is known as the

CHUNIN and their responsibilities include overseeing the education of the students, maintaining the morale of the clan high and tackling internal issues when they arise, if not resolved prior to.

Genin Field Agents

GENIN

Below the sub-commander, is the field operatives that are responsible for executing the clan's mission. Ninja operators are also known as GENIN. Field operatives comprise large proportions of the clan. their skills can vary between a young recruit to a veteran. The job of Genin Genin in the clan is vital. Their primary responsibility is to develop their abilities at all levels to ensure they can take on any challenge that comes their way. Genin can also be specialized in specific aspects in the field. Certain Genin are more skilled in concealment and stealth, while others are more knowledgeable of specific skills like poison making, reconnaissance or combat tactics.

THE DOJO

Dojo (training hall) Dojo (training Hall) is where all warriors gather to improve their skills by studying the practice, theory as well as application of martial arts which are administered through Kurai

Kotori Ryu. Kurai Kotori Ryu. It is believed that the Dojo is a place of spirituality that provides the warrior with a sanctuary from the rigors of everyday living. Once inside its walls the warrior is protected from outside chaos.

Dojo Dojo

The peace of the Dojo is evident in the warriors who study within its walls. The peace and tranquility of the Dojo allows freedom of development of the body, mind and soul.

As a hall of heroes like a hall of heroes, the Dojo draws its strength from those who are within. The strength and skill that the most skilled warriors of the clan sets the benchmark for the Dojo's strength and energy. The most skilled practitioners of the art are an example to the lower-ranking students, providing them with instructions during their studies. This is a major aspect of the Dojo environment. It is a space where veteran fighters freely share their knowledge with people who are just beginning their journey on the way of life.

Hall of Heroes

DOJO Uniform

The uniform used for training by students is a sturdy unidirectional black single-weave uniform which is extremely tough and is essential to withstand a lot of throwing and grappling. The uniform has an inside pocket that is located on the part of the part of the jacket. Also, the pant cuff is adorned with leg tie. Sleeves of this uniform have been cut to fit at the level of elbow. that left collar of the jacket has been decorated by the Kurai Kotori Crest.

Black Uniform

Leg Ties

Family Crest

MOUNTAIN SANCTUARY

When they can when they can, the warriors of Kurai Kotori clan train in a mountainous or wooded surroundings that resemble the hidden training facilities used by their ancient predecessors. As they hide in the natural environment, those who are part of the Kurai Kotori Ninjas are exposed details that aren't taught in the classroom. Skills like stealth and reconnaissance, infiltration, formations for battlefields trap deployment, in survival, and trap deployment. These are the abilities that are subject to studying while in the natural Dojo. This is a part is a part of Ninja instruction is built on experiences in contrast to the training that is conducted within the Dojo that is based on repetition. Only after experiencing the experience of being pursued by many shadows or becoming the warrior that sneaks into the camp of an adversary will one be able to comprehend the ability required to accomplish these tasks.

Mountain Sanctuary

CLASSICAL GARB

In the absence of the uniform for training that is in use in the Dojo and the Dojo's warriors from the Kurai Kotori clan wear the appropriate traditional garb that is worn by the Ninja and start exploring the dark corners. It is replaced by an obi-length (obi) sash (obi) with a split toe boots (tabi) are worn to enhance the sensitivity and stealth of the wearer and a shroud (zukin) is used to hide identity and conceal human forms and the Cloak (gaito) can be utilized to provide warmth and protection.

Classical Garb

Sash

Split Toe Shoes

Shroud

Cloak

Training STUCTURE

The structure of training in the Kurai Kotori Clan is comprised of three stages distinct from each other. The three stages are referred to informally as the Shoden (beginning phase) and The Chuden (advanced phase) along with Hiden (secret stage). Hiden (secret level). In these three stages, there are various levels of training which students are exposed to. Through being able to pass the mental and physical tests that are administered by the various levels that a student is able to acquire the skills and knowledge required to continue their learning. The third and final levels are an Okuden (verbal transmittal) part that is part of this art. These are enlightening teachings on subjects that are both inside and outside of the set course of training.

TITLES AND RANKING

While rank belts weren't employed in traditional Japanese system, they have a purpose showing a student's status on the way. Instead of an all-color belt system, it is the Kurai Kotori family has chosen an exclusive belt rank that every student receives the black belt when they join the school. The belt will be in the student's possession throughout their studies, the only thing that changes is the small colored stripe at the tip of the belt to show their rank. As they progress in rank, the stripe that was colored previously will be removed and replaced with an additional color to indicate the progress. Each rank is accompanied by an official title, which further indicates that they are in the direction.

TRANSLATION OF LEVEL TITLE RANK

SHODEN Shoshinsha Initiate Black Belt

1 White Stripe

SHODEN Chi Gakusei Earth

Student Black Belt

1 Red Stripe

SHODEN Sui Gakusei Water

Student Black Belt

1 Orange Stripe

SHODEN Ka Gakusei Fire

Student Black Belt

1 Yellow Stripe

SHODEN Fu Gakusei Wind

Student Black Belt

1 Green Stripe

CHUDEN Ku Yushi Celestial

Warrior Black Belt

1 Blue Stripe

CHUDEN Tashi Ninja

Master Black Belt

2 Blue Stripes

CHUDEN Renshi Refined

Master Black Belt

3 Blue Stripes

HIDEN Shinobi Ninja

Black Black Belt

4 Blue Stripes

HIDEN Shinobi Shujin Ninja

Master Black Belt

5 Blue Stripes

HIDEN Shinobi Meijin Ninja

Lord Black Belt

6 Blue Stripes

OKUDEN Seishin Shugisha Ninja

Spiritualist Black Belt

Blue Border

OKUDEN Tetsujin Ninja

Philosopher Black Belt

Silver Border

OKUDEN Kenja Ninja

Sage Black Belt

Gold Border

SUB-ARTS & PRIMARY ARTS

It is believed that the Kurai Kotori Tradition is a vast system with more than 30 Primary Arts , which house over 150 Sub-Arts, giving it the most thorough style of its kind in the world. The entire system could be a life-long journey that offers knowledge that is unique to all practitioners. Every person who follows the path has a unique skill set in different fields and ultimately develop an art form that is specialized according to their strengths and preferences to make an individual warrior.

A PARTIAL LIST SKILLS

The following is a graphic depiction of some of the techniques that compose the many facets in the art of Ninja.

ACROBATICS

Ninja are taught how to improve their body's flexibility through the use of a variety of specific drills and techniques. Taiso (calisthenics), Tai Sabaki (movement), Hakari (balance) Ukemi (breakfalls), Kaiten (rolls), Tobi (leaps), Tetobidasu (handsprings) along with Kuki Kaiten (aerial turns) are all studied in order to increase speed and agility until they reach an advanced level. These abilities can then be used as an addition to unarmed and armed combat, by using maneuvers in attack and defense as well as useful for climbs, stealth and concealment.

UNARMED COMBAT

Kurai Kotori Taijutsu (body practice) is inspired by the five elemental powers of water, earth winds, fire, and celestial. From the four main elements that comprise the Ninja learns to apply strategies for fighting that utilize the power of (earth) as well as cunning (water) as well as determination (fire) as well as agility (wind). When he develops these four qualities in equal measure as a team, the Ninja develops the capacity to adapt to the situation by permitting the most efficient element to come out whenever needed (celestial). The system of unarmed combat is well-informed about vital areas of attack (genkotsu) and muscle attacks (koshiwaza) and bone attack (koppowaza) and joints manipulation (kansetsuwaza) and throws (nagewaza) and tension attacks (gatamewaza) and fingers locks (yubiwaza) as well as constrictions attacks (shimewaza) as well as reverses (nukewaza) and defense against firearms (muto).

SWORDSMANSHIP

Skills with the sword are at the heart of the weaponry education for an Ninja. Training using swords like the Ninja sword (Shinobigatana) improves hand-eye coordination as well as improves the ability of a Ninja to discern the vital ability to judge timing, as well as distancing in combat. The Ninja sword was made to be practical and focuses on practicality over aesthetics. A blade that is shorter for greater speed and concealment with a hilt that is longer for an increased leverage as well as a bigger handguard with a square shape for better security. Apart from its evident cutting and striking abilities it is also a Ninja sword is also equipped with many subtle capabilities that boost its power. A robust scabbard is an additional weapon, as well as a storage container where blinding powder that can be sprayed in the eye of a foe and a cord could be used to tie or shake the scabbard.

FOUR ESSENTIAL WEAPONS

There are four weapons that provide the foundation of all weapons training. Hanbo (short staff) is a method of teaching using STICK weapons that are based on STICK, which is defined as any weapon that is solid and does not is focused on striking and thrusting and methods of locking joints while grappling. Tanto (dagger) is a teacher of the usage of BLADE weaponry, which is which is defined as having an edge that cuts or a sharp point that emphasizes stabbing and slashing, as well as the techniques for using the pommel. Kusari Fundo (short chain) will teach the use of FLEXIBLE weapons that are which is defined as anything with flexible nature, which emphasizes flailing, as well as a variety of ways of connecting. Kusari Fundo (short chain) is a form of entanglement Kugi (spikes) teach the use of PROJECTILE-based weapons, which are defined as anything that is able to be shot or thrown, and that focuses on stabbing or striking and also methods of attack using pressure points when grappling.

SHURIKENJUTSU - TWISTING BLADES

Throwing blades goes long before the time of the past of Japan when a royal warrior launched an attack by throwing the Hashi (chopsticks) into his opponent. The method proved extremely effective and has been referred to as "Shurikenjutsu," which translates to "The blade that is behind the hands," which means that the throwing device should only be employed to create a sense of surprise, either to gain the initiative or secure escape. Very rarely has a shuriken been acknowledged as killing the enemy or a person, and even in those cases where there was a death the cause was probably caused by a lethal layer of poison, not the weapon itself. It is believed that the Kurai Kotori Ninja has a variety of throwing blades, but those with a cross (juji) quarter moon (hangetsu) as well as the spike (kugi) and the four-pointed (shippo) are the most popular. Beyond weapons that are specifically designed to be to be thrown at, the Ninja can transform almost everything into an explosive projectile.

STAVES and CLUBS

Bojutsu (staff combat) is a form of combat using poles made of bamboo, wood or rattan with various lengths. The Bojutsu art is comprised of an array of powerful bludgeoning tools. Larger weapons, such as Hammer (kanazuchi) studded staff (konsaibo) iron staff (tetsubo) and the oar (kai) and the mace (tsuchiboko) are highly efficient in battle scenarios. In close-range scenarios weapons such as iron fan (tesson) the iron truncheon (jutte) spin rods (shobo) small sticks (hananegi) as well as the hand stick (kobo) the iron fist (tekkon) as well as the fighting rings (bankokuchoki) along with forearms, the shinguards (kote as well as sune) and shields (kame) can be more efficient. These and other strike weapons give with the Ninja with the capability to deliver blunt trauma hits which can break bones and inflict concussive harm to opponents.

HALBERDS

While the sword is a powerful weapon however, the halberd proved itself to be more effective in battlefield battles. It is the Kurai Kotori Ninja utilizes three principal styles. Straight edged halberd (nagimaki) as well as the curly bladed halberd (naginata) as well as the halberd with a heavy blade (bisento). They were created to ensure to ensure that it was possible for the Ninja could still utilize fluid sword-like movements while staying at a distance that was safer, which is the primary purpose in any kind of weapon, be it spear, staff, or halberd. If used correctly the weapons can dominate any battle that allows the user to concentrate more on offensive moves and less on defensive strategies. One powerful blow could break limbs and destroy armor.

CHAILS AND FLAILS

Chains and flails are incredibly useful due to their concealability, as well as their efficiency when used to strike, flail and/or create entanglements. When properly flailed the weighted end can gain massive momentum, which generates a tremendous power that could shatter bones. The main weapon in this system is an 6' - to 9' chain that is weighted (o-kusari). It is extremely effective against swordsmen due to the length of the chain allows the wearer to remain outside the reach of the blade , while the weighted end of the chain is placed against the wrists of swordsmen. The O-kusari is generally flailed to keep the opponent at bay. When an opening is created it is whipped into attack. Other weapons are the chain and ball (gekigan) chain whip (muchi Kusari) and chain bola (san Kusari) as well as the sickle chain (nagegama) as well as the two-sectional flail (ni setsu kon) and the three-sectional flail (san setsu kon).

SICKLES AND AXES

Twin sickles (nichogama) are a devastating tool. Their strength lies in their capability to confuse an opponent by presenting an infinite array of hypnotic moves, and the fact that they can be employed in pairs, which allows one to attack as other attack, giving Ninjas Ninja an ability to employ offensive and defensive methods simultaneously. Because blades are connected with the shafts on these weapon, they're also capable of intricate methods of traps and manipulation. Other weapons used in mid-range within the system include deeply curving sickles (natagama) smaller sickles (kogama) twin axes (masakari) and the an axe (te ono). There are two more powerful weapons that are taught in the kamajutsu technique. A great sickle (ogama) and the great the axe (o-no) two of which are weighty and bulky to be used in pairs.

SPEAR

Being the victim of a properly directed spear thrust is like receiving poisonous poison. This is due to the fact that the three-sided spear (sankakuyari) features a unique made triangular blade which causes wounds that are not closed which means that even minor of injuries cause the death of a patient because of the constant loss of blood. In addition to an triangular bladed style there are a variety of spear designs utilized for the Ninja. The hook-bladed spear (kamayari) was created to catch and hold the enemy's weapon as well as legs. The spear's blades are open (hokoyari) is akin to the inside of the crescent moon. Pendulum spear (furikoyari) features an elongated blade capable of unleashing powerful broad-based attacks. The spear with a short blade (shakujoyari) includes the shaft which is strengthened like a staff, and a tiny double edged blade which is utilized for swift cutting and thrusts.

CORDS and CORDS AND

The little-known method of using nets and cords can be extremely useful for the Ninja operating. The primary reason why these weapons are so effective is their ability to be concealed. Although they seem to be less powerful as other guns, it only helps make their impressive whipping and trapping methods more enthralling. They are equipped with the capability to tie arms, disarm weapons and make breath constrict. They are the ultimate tool for silent elimination. The main weapon used of the system, the silken rope (torinawa) which is utilized to tie and restrain an adversary. The other weapons are the huge net (o-toami) carried by one or two Ninja and the smaller net (chu-toami) which is utilized by one Ninja and it is the net whip (muchi-toami) which is used as a complement weapon to either a short spear or a sword and the rope as well as a hook (kaginawa) employed in combat as well as for climbing.

BOW AND BOW AND

The bow and arrow were some of the first guns used for military use of Japan. Kyubajutsu (the method used by bows and horses) is described in several of Japan's oldest historical texts. At the beginning the bow and arrow were primarily used to defend to Kyubasen (mounted archers) and Tohosen (foot archers) in firing at enemies in close proximity. However, later on, archers took on an edgier position shooting their bows in a volley style, producing a flood of shafts with razor-tipped tips. One of the main aspects that has remained same with the art of Hankyu (short bow) is discipline. Only those who have the ability to maintain calm and unwavering determination are thought to have the ability to shoot an arrow under the guidance of a god. Another weapon within the system is called the crossbow (jujikakyu).

DARTS AND BLOWGUNS

Shotguns (fukidake) or darts (fukiya) are two of the Ninja's preferred tactics for tackling enemies. A properly placed shot can deliver deadly doses of poison in the blood stream of an unwary target or hinder a chaser or cause a horse of an adversary to rear when struck by an invisible projectile. The reason it is a weapon of choice is because the Ninja is not required to fight a skilled opponent directly. It is not worth risking a loss in the hands of an armored and superiorly armed adversary when a tiny air-guided missile can be fired from a distance. The art of shooting is often coupled with the ability to create animal, plant or artificial poisons (dokujutsu).

COMBINATION WEAPONS

The world of Ninjutsu there are many tools that require two or more weapons skills. For example, the Kyoketsushayoge (rope knife) is a weapon which consists of an axe (tanto) and a hook blade (kama) and rope (torinawa) as well as a large metal rings (bankokuchoki). It is also known as the Kusarigama (sickle with chain) is a weapon that combines the deadly close-range sickle (kama) along with a long chain with a weighted weight (kusari) for a weapon with multiple ranges. Other weapons that can be combined include the chain and short staff (chigiriki) along with a flail and staff (bo the karazao) and staffs equipped with a concealed chain (feruzue) and staffs that have a the blade concealed (shikomizue). Each of these weapons should be examined in detail before they are able to be effectively used. This way, the soldier is aware of each weapon's advantages and disadvantages, and allows them to utilize each weapon to its maximum potential when used together.

SWORD RESTRAINMENT WEAPONS

The sword, as the primary weapon used by the Japanese warrior caste, offered the Ninja with a fascinating problem. The challenge was to develop weapons that could limit or limit a swordsman's capability to engage in combat. While each of the Ninja's primary weapons were able to provide effective self-defense however, it was the creation of tools for restraint which greatly enhanced effectiveness of their weapons to protect against the lightning-fast knife from the Samurai. The most specialized weapons included the iron truncheon (jutte) as well as the man-catcher (sasumata) and T-staff (tsukabo) and sleeve entangler (sodegarami) and the tiger claws (torashuko) However there are many other specific tools that made it possible to exploit flaws in the deadly weapon of the Samurai and armor.

HIDDEN WEAPONS

Hidden weapons are the most sought-after Ninja particularity. Making use of everyday objects as weapons or concealing secrets devices that could later be used against an enemy requires a keen sense of shrewdness and strategic thinking. A well-hidden weapon is visible but is not a threat to the person who is observing it. In this regard it is no surprise that the Kurai Kotori Ninja embark on their quest to create weapons that are almost invisible, like the spiked rings (kakute) poison needle (dokubari) Garrote (nawa fundo) wood comb (kushi) as well as a the folding fan (senssu) the blinding powder (metsubishi) umbrella (kasa) cats claws (nekote) Clogs made of wood (geta) chopsticks (hashi) prayers beads (juzu) and sash (obi) and many more tools that are improvised.

Firearms and CANNONS

A Ninja's use explosives and fire is a legend. Inhaling an erupting cloud of smoke or using explosions that cause damage are just a few of the Ninja's best tactics. Ninja employed these tactics since the time they obtained the right chemicals from the Mongols at the end of the 1200's. It is no surprise that the Ninja would be a fan of cannons and firearms when they were made available in the mid 1500's. The barrel's length affected the precision and accuracy of the firearm. While a musket with a long barrel (jozutsu) could be more effective in sniping weapons at far distances however, the Ninja typically preferred shorter muzzles (chuzutsu) or handguns of smaller size (tanzutsu) to have more intimate encounters. In addition to these guns they also had handguns. Ninja also produced hand guns (sodezutsu) which were not extremely accurate however they had blasts that were large and they were effective against more than one opponent at one time.

Stealth

There is a popular belief there is a belief that the Ninja is the ultimate master of stealth. They are able to disappear at will or transform into wild animal form to vanish. Actually, it's Ninja's knowledge of invisibility which gives them an advantage. In reality, invisibility is understanding how to fool enemies ' senses so that they remain invisible, similar to how magicians manipulate their senses to confuse and confuse. To achieve this feat they must Ninja must master specialized techniques of movement that are quiet (kage-aruki) and running (hayagakejutsu) and crawling (hofukujutsu) as well as creating false noises (gionjutsu) and also using animals that have been trained (dobutsujutsu) and an understanding of the human perception. In addition to these abilities they need to know that a Ninja must be mentally ready to maintain an unremarkable, quiet brain (kage-shin) to conceal their motives.

CONCEALMENT

Even though the majority of Ninja are trained to be stealthy and adept at invisibility techniques There is always the chance that they'll be spotted. In this scenario, the Ninja should be able to effectively conceal. The techniques used to conceal are inspired by earth (chigakure) using the use of dirt, rocks and artificial structures. Water (suigakure) is made up of ponds, streams, or lakes. Fire (kagakure) made use of flame, light smoke, and explosives. Wind (kazegakure) makes use of snow, wind fog, rain, and wind. Perhaps the final and most efficient, Celestial (hensogakure), using everything that could alter the image of the Ninja to make them disappear from view by taking on the appearance and characteristics of a the person who is more likely to not be noticed.

Escape

The Ninja must research their adversaries' strategists and leaders in order to discover what kind of battlefield strategies they're most likely to encounter during their journey. If they think this way it is possible for the Ninja can come up with a variety of escape strategies that are actually counter to the strategies used by the soldiers of the enemy. This gives an Ninja with the capability to remain just one step in front of adversaries. Avoiding terrain that tracks making traps, concealing caches for supplies and weapons and luring enemies to ambushes planned for them are all effective strategies. It could take months to study the activities of the adversaries before the Ninja is able to recognize patterns in their actions However, the length of time spent isn't important. In the final analysis the Ninja will be able to know more regarding the adversary than they is aware of themselves.

RECONNAISSANCE AND INFILTRATION

In the intricate art of reconnaissance (teisatsujutsu) and infiltration (sennyujutsu) the Ninja learns to search out enemy fortifications learn their strengths and weakness, learn the layout and gather information from the locals, and relay that information and any other relevant information on to clan members. Ninja reconnaissance teams are utilized to identify possible battlefields well before any battle was scheduled to be fought. They then provide an extensive map of every one of the terrain contours, which would provide some light on how troops could best be placed. Infiltrating an area or structure The Ninja must be aware of the schedule of every person operating within the zone of target and the zones with the least traffic, physical obstacles that block their way, as well as if there are any allies who could be recruited to help.

SURVIVAL Skills

Seizonjutsu one of the ways to survive, has paramount importance for the Ninja. Being able to survive in the wild was not an option, it was a requirement. A majority of Ninja were able to conduct their operations in distant mountain and forest areas to ensure they were in the shadows of those who would resist their activities. Being in such a hostile environment created Ninja extremely tough and resilient. It is essential to have the proper clothes, water sources ability to build fires as well as a grasp of the concept of makeshift shelters cutting tools, a illumination, non-perishable foodstuffs creation knowing about the resources of animals and plants, and setting up the base camp in a secure area with feasible escape routes.

GROUP TACTICS

Group tactics (senjojutsu) is an important component of combative actions. The training helps the skills of a Ninja in many ways particularly in the area of collaboration. Senjojutsu tactics are generally used in a striking force comprising between five and seven Ninja. Though small by the standards of battlefield warfare, these top teams are extremely effective in accomplishing a range of tasks without being detected. Therefore, highlighting that stealth is more effective than engaging in direct combat with enemies. The challenges a team will face on the field are endless, and the team has to be constantly tested through simulations of missions in order to sharpen their reflexes to the highest level. Each of the Ninja team members have specific skills, tools and equipment that make them more efficient together.

ESPIONAGE TACTICS

Being able to manipulate the environment around them is essential ingredient to becoming a highly effective agent. An effective Ninja is required to assess their adversaries' character in a moment's notice to identify vulnerabilities that could be exploited. The same analysis process applied to the surroundings within which the enemy operates is applicable. Once the Ninja is aware of their adversaries and their strengths, they can create events that trigger the enemy to act as the Ninja desires without even realizing, and even when they do the truth, it's probably too for them to do anything to change the situation. Making false connections, recruiting as pawns, encouraging betrayal among allies, and releasing fake information or actions that cause the enemy to be entangled in the web of illusion created by the Ninja.

PSYCHOLOGICAL WARFARE

The Ninja is a mental fighter as a physical one. The Ninja is an apparition in the enemy's mind. In the end, the Ninja is looking for any mental weakness in their opponent which can be exploited. If there are no weaknesses to be found then the Ninja will make one up for them by the use of specific methods of manipulation in the mind called Saiminjutsu or The technique of using hypnosis. A Ninja must be able to master the spectre of the mind tactic, without divulging their motives. The adversary should be completely ignorant of any manipulation until it's too far gone. In earlier times, Ninja were often depicted as being in a relationship with demon forces that caused their enemies to think of them as being supernatural.

MYSTICISM

Gorin Kuji Myo Himitsu Shaku The Secret Wisdom of Inner Strength uses deep meditation techniques designed to awaken the hidden spiritual abilities that reside deep within each Ninja. If the Ninja is able to harness their inner strength they will be able to accomplish extraordinary feats. Techniques like increasing physical and mental power, healing capabilities and directing spiritual energy projecting emotions and thoughts and reaching into the shadow. As eerie as it sounds the power is present in all human beings. They aren't magical powers but rather personal spiritual energy which, if focused can result in the development of extraordinary abilities that transcend the boundaries of human capabilities.

THEATRICAL COMBAT

Chambara refers to the Japanese name for a distinct type of action film that celebrated Japan's Feudal period. The thing that made these films distinct is that they didn't just told interesting stories but also kept a realistic fighting. The skills of combat were not faked using sophisticated camera techniques since actors were skilled fighters of swordsmanship. The skills shown on screen did not have any connection to the modern styles of competitive fighting in the present, but were based on the highly effective combative art which were solely designed for the effective elimination of an adversaries. The films of the time were the ideal way to tell stories of the heroic adventures of the mighty Samurai as well as the unrequited and tragic path of masterless Ronin as well as the deceitful and enigmatic actions that were performed by the ghostly Ninja. A lot of Kurai Kotori Ninjutsu practitioners are Chambara artists.

Modern technology

Mirai Shinobi, also known as Future Ninja, is a word that describes the Ninja with a background in martial arts, but also adept using modern weapons and techniques. Rifles, handguns smoke grenades, Tasers, liquid-eye irritants as well as restraint devices such as the body armour, tools and surveillance equipment, lock pickers, and everything else that is available in our modern times that is seamlessly integrated into Ninja's primary art.

Chapter 9: Etiquette

Reishiki also known as "Etiquette," is a vital aspect of martial instruction. For those who aren't familiar with the subject, Reishiki appears to be an approach to make students submit to their instructors. But, the practice of etiquette within the Dojo does not have anything to do with these things. Reishiki can be used to structure the dojo into an effective society, showing the discipline, dedication as well as common sense and of course, good manners.

TRANSLATION

Reishiki is derived in the two Japanese words. The first word is "Rei" and is defined by bow salutation, salute property, courtesy ceremony, thanks and gratitude. The second component of the phrase refers to "Shiki" and is said to mean ceremony, rite , or function. Together, the term "Reishiki" is translated as ceremony, ritual or ceremonial behavior.

EASTERN THOUGHT/WESTERN EYES

To an Westerner Reishiki may appear to be a strange phenomenon However, a more thorough examination is necessary to fully comprehend the significance. Some ask "What does this whole ritual have got to do with teaching how to fight?" The answer to that is ....everything. The primary goal for Reishiki is to put the mind in a healthy state to be taught more effectively how to be a better learner.

The essence of REISHIKI

While a student is in training, Reishiki takes on important and increasingly more important functions. It is a fundamental component of Shugyo (warrior cultivation). It tests the student's ability to surrender their self-esteem to the whims of destruction. In this way, it is the base that is used to temper the spirit of the warrior. However, we do not really destroy the ego of a student. Instead, we try to polish and mould the student's ego by putting them through challenges, hardships and reflection.

SELF-SACRIFICE

The acceptance or rejection of Reishiki can be used to reveal a student's devotion or inadequacies to the Sensei (teacher). A student who is constantly questioning or is unable to accept Reishiki isn't a good candidate to continue their training as they view their personal views and opinions in a way that is superior to goals and goals of Ryu. Distracted by their own self-absorption one who disrespects Reishiki is unable to accept reality that the obligation as a learner is primarily towards Reishiki, the Ryu (clan) as well as the good of others over their own.

ETIQUETTE BREEDS SUCCESSFUL

The experience gained through Reishiki together with the technique of executing the techniques of the Ryu are combined into one unique expression. The combination of both physical and mental experiences eventually change the soul. The greater sensitivity that comes from the ongoing cultivation of warriors lets the student peer into their own soul in a way that they have never seen before. This is an epiphany sort for many. It is a moment when responsibility to the Ryu as well as their elders as well as to humanity in general becomes more significant than satisfying their own desires. Thus, a generous spirit is developed and the ability to think is allowed to thrive. The abstract concepts of death and life place the existence of the student in its appropriate natural setting. The transcendence of the spirit realm frequently appears as a first-time experience. Through the years of studying, the student's identity, he becomes one with the world, and to the realm in which those spirits from our ancestors dwell. In the absence of this sensitivity and growing awareness of their position in the world martial artists can be lost and end up with untrue moral codes which justifies the ego-driven desire for self-gratification and justified violence. The knowledge gained from proper Reishiki protects you from Kam I which are "deities" to ward off the evil that mankind has been fighting for centuries. The evil that is causing the most harm is violence of a malevolent nature and a curse that has become the bane of our existence.

ETIQUETTE GUIDELINES

Students should be sure to learn the guidelines for etiquette. These guidelines serve as the basis of how you can be a part of the Kurai Kotori clan conducts itself in the training setting and students must follow the rules with diligence.

DOJO ENTRY

1. Make sure you arrive on time for training. If you consistently arrive absent without reason, it's inexcusable.

2. After entering the Dojo students must take off their shoes prior to moving to the area for training.

Outdoor footwear is not allowed on the training floor.

3. As you enter or exit the Dojo students should always bow to toward the Kamiza (dojo Shrine) part at the back of the Dojo. If there's no shrine, bow instead as they enter and exit the doorway.

4. Be sure to greet the instructor upon first arrive for your training session so that they know that have arrived and are ready to learn.

5. The most common phrase you hear when meeting your teacher can be "Osu!" In Japanese the word"Osu" is made up by two letters. First, the character described by the term "Push." Its second is described by the term "Endure." It's commonly used to show reverence and may be used to substitute phrases and words like "yes," "all right," "good," "I will try,"" "I will give it my best," and "excuse me." In actual fact, students are expected to not even ever "Hello" to his teachers and instead use the phrase "OSU" in lieu. In its purest form, it's an appeal to one's self to conquer the flaws of the human condition. One word is the philosophy behind Ninjutsu. The ideal student must have"the "Spirit of Osu." This is the primary force behind the tradition that affects the Ninja practitioner's performance of their obligations, physical training, and interactions with others.

UNFORMATION AND EQUIPMENT

1. All uniforms should be correctly tailored. Sleeves should be cut approximately below elbow. The pants are secured to the calf area with leg tie. A family name (patch) is placed on the left side of the chest over the heart. It is essential to keep uniforms clear of wrinkles and kept clean.

2. Dressing room manners - Black belts and the upper ranks should be permitted to change their clothes first at the conclusion of the class. Students with lower rank should wait in silence outside their respective dressing rooms to wait for their turn. Do not put anything away in the dressing rooms. Students must bring their equipment in the Dojo and then take their equipment to home according to the class.

3. Students should not wear their tie belts or leg ties at the Dojo. The items must be removed before leaving in the locker room.

4. All equipment such as training weapons, safety equipment and armor, as well as any other equipment that is used for training must be purchased through Dojo sources.

5. The student is accountable for all the weapons and equipment needed according to their grade. It is not the responsibility of Dojo to provide these items. Dojo is not in charge of providing these tools for use by students. If a student continues to show in the Dojo without the proper equipment and equipment, they won't be allowed to participate.

Always be prepared with the most basic weaponry and tools

PREPAREMENT for TRAINING

1. It is not recommended to do any practice that is not supervised prior to class, so that students don't need to be cautious while moving into and out of the locker rooms. The practice of, particularly weapons, without being told to do so is extremely inconsiderate.

2. After changing after changing, the student must sit at the side, armed using the proper training equipment and sit down until the beginning of class. Alternatively, they can begin some gentle stretching to prepare the body for the training.

3. While in the Dojo students should not ever lean on their weapons or lean against the wall. This is an obvious sign of indifference. Be tall and aware to the information being provided.

4. There are two methods to sit in the Dojo. One is to be with the "Seiza," or "Kneeling" Position. The other is to sit at a "Fudoza," or "Cross-legged" position. Don't lie down to the ground, unless injured.

5. If the instruction "Seiretsu" is issued to all students, they must align themselves in front of the Kamiza in order of the rank of the student. (If the sword is employed, it is carried by the scabbard of the right hand, just beneath the

guard. The pommel should point towards the rear and the blade will tip forward, the cutting the edge downwards).

6. If the instruction "Sabate" is given, all students must be required to kneel in a Seiza position. (If swords are being utilized, it will be placed on the right side of the student with the pommel facing forward and cutting the edge inwards).

7. If the command "Sensei ni rei" is issued, all students should put their right hand on the ground in front of them , followed with their left. The fingers on the pointer of each hand must be in contact with their thumbs to create an opening in the triangle between hands. The student bows forward. The teacher returns the bow. Students cannot be allowed to rise until the teacher is up out of their bow. When the student is up the left hand of their teacher is placed in their lap, followed by their right.

8. The teacher will then toward the Kamiza. If the instruction "Zarei" is spoken teachers and pupils will bow towards the Kamiza. Students will not lift from their bows until the teacher has risen. (If there is a sword being employed, it must be placed directly in front of the pupil prior to bowing, with the pommel facing to the left and cutting edge to the left).

9. When the instruction "Mokuso" is announced students are instructed to place their left hand in the palm of the right hand, and turn their eyes away to meditate in a quiet place.

Quiet Thought

10. After a few minutes in silence, instructor will get up to a sitting position and then turn his back to the students.

11. If the instruction "Sodachi" is issued students will be raised to a standing posture. To stand correctly it is necessary to begin by lowering their feet until their toes touch the ground under their hips. The student then lifts their right leg towards the right side, and use it to pull their body into an upright position. (If there is a sword being utilized, the student should hold it in their right hand underneath the guard and then lift the sword up to a vertical position by their side while they climb. After standing, the weapon is moved to the left hand and placed horizontally on the waist or tucked into the belt).

12. If the instruction "Gasso" is given, both the teacher and students should place their hands together with their palms in the front of their chests and then bow to the waist. (If the sword is employed, the student must keep their position

on their left, and move their right hand up to salute).

DURING the course of training.

1. It is crucial to inform your instructor of any physical ailments you may be suffering from prior to starting your training. If the injury is serious it is recommended that a red cloth is tied to the affected limb to ensure the other students and instructors are reminded not to touch the location. When the issue is located on the upper torso, the strip cloth could be tied to the belt.

2. . If you have to go home before the end of class, ensure that you inform the instructor know in advance that you have to quit early. You must bow to your teacher then bow to your partner and walk out of the classroom. Dress yourself and walk away quietly and be sure to not disturb other students. It's not a good idea to consistently be late to class or leave before being officially dismissed.

3. If you are training on your own (tandoku Renshu) or when the entire class is in a line to perform striking drills, acrobatics and footwork exercises or any other single-person activity instructors will start by yelling "Yoi!" or "Ready!" Students will respond by saying "Yosh!" in a highly focused and focused tone. In the majority of cases, these drills are performed in groups of 10.

After the tenth movement the student needs to perform a loud "Kiai!".

4. When an instructor exhibits the technique or shows any additives or variables, students should pay attention and observe. If asked to complete the instruction, the students must respond by saying "Hai!" or "Yes!" Another acceptable response is "Osu!"

5. If two students play with each other (sotai Renshu) there always will be a defense (Tori) as well as an attacker (Uke). The Uke will take an aggressive stance as the Tori will react by executing preplanned strategies designed to stop the attack. The relationship between the two students is one of cooperation not competition. Uke does not intend to hurt Tori The goal is to assist Tori improve her skills through repetition of techniques. The partnership is one of mutual respect. In groups in a group, the top student is Tori (defender) and the next highest ranking taking on the job that of Uke (attacker).

6. If joints are locked, thrown, or other techniques to immobilize the body are used, the possibility of physical discomfort should be anticipated. The appropriate reaction is to ask Uke to touch the floor using their hands in a manner that shows that the technique is working. If hands aren't at a level to be tapped, the phrase "Itai!" or "It hurts!" is an appropriate response. If

you get injured, inform the instructor know right away and they will take care of the incident. Students should continue to train unless they are required to assist the injured.

Tori (defender) is able to stop an attack after Uke (attacker) presses

7. Uke must not attempt to interfere with or interfere with Tori's technique, unless explicitly instructed to take action. A teacher might ask Uke to provide different amounts of resistance Tori to assist in testing the ability of Tori to use the technique.

8. In some instances, students will be allowed to fight in the open (jiyu Renshu) in controlled striking or grappling competitions. They could pit one person against another, one with several opponents or even two or more students against many opponents. These games are designed to illustrate the fact that the situation can change in a moment's notice. the ability of a student to adapt to change will decide the outcome. Tori (defender) ends the technique once Uke (attacker) strikes the 132 effectiveness in physical fight. There should be no sparring or any other type of partner training without an instructor who is supervising.

9. . It is the Dojo headmaster (Jonin) is in the Dojo for a reason to teach. It is the duty of the student to sit in the ground and sit down waiting for Jonin to answer their questions. In this way, there is no conflict in instruction. The fact that a student is the rank of a black belt, it is not a guarantee that they will be an option for less ranked students. Jonin will determine if other black belts should be used in the teaching process.

After training

1. If class has come to an over...it's finished. Students are not allowed to practice practicing without supervision after class. If you're blessed with excessive energy, you must tidy the Dojo to make it ready for the next day's training.

2. It is the responsibility of the student to maintain the Dojo clean and tidy. If the trash bin is overflowing and you have to empty it, do so. If mats are in need of cleaning take them off, and if the floor is filthy, sweep it. The Dojo is your reflection and a messy Dojo indicates that its members are uncaring and lazy. It's not a duty but an honor to be able to learn the art of the warrior, therefore ensure it is maintained with respect and care.

Cleaning the Dojo

AT SOCIAL EVENTS

1. Etiquette isn't just limited to training in a dojo. Your instructor is your instructor, regardless of the location.

Guest Instructors

1. Whatever the their style or affiliation, every instructor that is hired to instruct students must be treated with the utmost respect. They might have taken an alternative route, but their commitment and effort are worthy of admiration.

LEADERSHIP / TEACHING CREDIT

1. Credentials for teaching are granted to students who have studied the principles and practice of the techniques and skills that are taught in the Kurai Kotori Clan, and have obtained Black Belt III (Renshi). Candidates who have earned this accreditation are required to keep the open lines of communications with Hombu Dojo in an honest determination to be current on any modifications or additions to the structure of training. In the absence of this, it invalidates the instructor's right to be a representative of the art.

2. Instructors who are certified should continue their own professional development by regularly visiting at least once a year the Hombu Dojo or having the Jonin visit their school or location at least every year. While not required the visits are essential to continue growth.

3. Training sessions will have a thorough attention to Unarmed Combat, Acrobatics, Basic Swordsmanship and Weaponry. These four abilities are thought of as to be the basis of the Kurai Kotori system.

4. Specific skills that involve Advanced Weapons, Stealth, Mysticism, Invisibility and others... can be learned in specially designed training courses with deadline-sensitive goals to complete the task.

5. Any instructor, regardless of rank is allowed to take it upon them to modify any training material, either in verbal or written form without written permission. Any changes made to the clan structure are approved by Hombu Dojo and it is the instructor's responsibility to keep them in place.

6. Any instructor with a certification can teach an individual, however, all rank advancements are given from the Kurai Kotori Martial Arts Federation under the authority of Jonin. Jonin.

7. Every instructor will supply them with one of their patches that bear the clan kamon . These patches are sewn on your left side of the uniform. The clan kamon is the only logo or image that is more important than the clan symbol.

8. Training materials cannot be developed and distributed without prior prior written consent

from Hombu Dojo. Hombu Dojo. All pertinent material will be made available through Hombu Dojo. Hombu Dojo. Training materials will be given a version number and date, so that it is easy to track updates.

TERMINOLOGY

The ability to understand terminology is crucial in understanding the art of. A lot of Japanese alphabets sound the same the way they sound in English However, some letters are written and spoken differently.

Japanese Sound English Sound Example

A AH (as the father) an ah, as in father. (ah-ka)

ai i (as in eye) Kurai (Koo-rai)

e ei (as in ray) Yame (yah-may)

ei ay (as in day) Sensei (sehn-say)

i ee (as in key) Jonin (joh-neen)

o oh (as in go) Dojo (doh-joh)

Oi"oy" (as in toys)"Yoi" (yoy)

U oo (as as in the"boot) Ninjutsu (nin-joot-soo)

tsu too (as in the near future) Tsuki (soo-key)

THE CLAN / ARTS

1. Kurai Kotori Ryu Kurai Kotori Ryu Clan of the Dark Lone Bird

2. Ninjutsu- Art of the Ninja

3. Kenjutsu -- Art of the Sword

4. Chambara -- Art of Theatrical Combat

TITLES/POSITIONS

1. Jonin - Leader / Headmaster

2. Jiki Deshi - Direct Apprentice

3. Kenshi - Sword master

4. Sensei - Teacher

5. Taisho General/Leader of the Dojo they own. Dojo

6. Chunin - Sub-commander / Organizer

7. Genin - Field Agent/ Student

UNIFORM or GARB

1. Mon - Family Crest

2. Hakama - Pleated skirt divided into pants

3. Keikogi - Training jacket

4. Shinobi Shozuku - Classical Ninja uniform

5. Zukin - Shroud / Hood

6. Tekoh - Forearm sleeves

7. Kyahan - Leg wraps

8. Tabi - Split toe shoes

9. Obi - Belt / Sash

10. Kimo - Cord / Leg Ties

11. Gaito - Cloak E

WEAPONS/EQUIPMENT

1. Katana - Long sword

2. Shinobigatana - Straight sword

3. Bokuto - A wooden sword

4. Chikuto Bamboo Sword

5. Hanbo 3 foot long staff

6. Tanto - Knife

7. Kusari Fundo - Weighted chain

8. Shaken Wheel - Bladed

9. Kugi throwing spikes

Training

1. Seiretsu - Line up

2. Sabate - Sit

3. Sensei Ni Rei - bow to teacher

4. Zarei - Spiritual bow

5. Mokuso Mokuso Quiet Thought 6. Sodachi"Stand Up"

7. Tori - Defender

8. Uke - Attacker

9. Yoi - Ready!

10. Kata - Forms prearranged

11. Waza - Technique prearranged

12. Ie - No

13. Hai Yes

14. Itai! It's hurting!

15. Yame - Stop

COUNTING

1. Ichi - One 16. Ju Roku - 16

2. Ni two 17. Jushichi Seventeen

3. San Three 18. Three 18. Ju hachi - Eighteen

4. Shi - Four 19. Ju ku - Nineteen

5. Go Five 20. Ni Ju - Twenty

6. Roku Six 21. Ni ju ichi

7. Shichi Seven

8. Hachi - Eight

9. Ku - Nine

10. Ju Ten Ten

11. Ju ichi - Eleven

12. Ju Ni Twelve

13. Ju San Thirteen

14. Ju shi - Fourteen

15. Ju go - Fifteen

16. Ju Roku 16

17. Jushichi 7teen

18. Ju hachi - Eighteen

19. Ju ku - Nineteen

20. Niju 20

21. Ni ju ichi

22. Niju nu

23. Niju su

24. Ni Ju Shi

25. Ni ju go

26. Ni Ju Roku

27. Ni Ju shichi

28. Ni ju hachi

29. Ni ju ku ku

30. San ju

DIRECTIONAL

1. Migi - Right

2. Hiadari - Left

3. Zenpo / Mae - Forward / Front

4. Koho / Ushiro - Back / Rear

5. Yoko Side

6. Naname - Naname -

7. Mawate - Turn

8. Omote - Outside

9. Ura Inside

CONVERSATIONAL

1. Domo Arigato Gozaimas - Thank you very much

2. Do Itashimashita - You're welcome

3. Ohayo - Good morning

4. Konnichiwa - Good afternoon

5. Konbanwa - Good evening

6. Oyasuminasai - Good night

7. Sayonara - Goodbye

Chapter 10: Virtues Laws And Doctrines

Kurai Kotori Ninja Kurai Kotori Ninja follow the specific set of virtues as well as laws and doctrines which provide guidance on the way they handle their encounters throughout their lives. First , there are what are the Virtues of the Ninja. These virtues are the guidelines for how the Ninja is able to live their daily day. Following is The Laws of the Ninja. The laws assist the Ninja during times of conflict, and set the standards for how they handle adversaries. Then there are the doctrines that govern the Ninja. The doctrines focus on the inner functioning of the Ninja's existence . They can be used to help stimulate a deeper insight into the powers that determine one's destiny.

The NINJA VIRTUES

Six particular virtues the Ninja follows. These virtues help that Ninja how to handle familial, personal and clan situations.

GRI -- DUTY

Giri can be described best by the Ninja as his "Obligation" towards the Clan. There are no limitations for the Ninja's sacrifice. Even though it's extreme by American norms, Giri is maintained to ensure the prosperity of the clan. If Giri is part of the clan, the group will flourish.

Because the purpose of the clan is also the individual Ninja's goal too. In this way there is no limit to what can be achieved.

SHIKI - RESOLUTE

Shiki recommends that Ninja must be determined in achieving their goals, and willing to go through any inconvenience or humiliation to achieve their goals. If an Ninja embarks on a quest to accomplish something, they must never be able to fail.

FuDO Strength

The idea of Fudo is to say that the Ninja must have a strong mind and body. This is vital because any weakness, whether physical or mental, could be exploited by an adversary.

DORYO - MAGNANIMITY

Any person who has power must make wise use of it. This is the point that the Ninja should remember that possessing the capability to kill doesn't necessarily make it a good idea to use it. To be an authentic warrior, one needs to understand the significance of mercy.

ONSHA - GENEROSITY

To succeed on the road one needs to realize the importance of giving. Making use of one's abilities to help others is truly honourable. Being selfless in words and deeds not only gives honour to the Ninja as well as the clan they represent.

NINYO (NINYO) CHIVALROUS

Ninyo stipulates that whenever conflicts arise there is a conflict, the Ninja must not be afraid to take action. This is the moment that the Ninja must determine what justifies using their abilities when they interfere in the affairs of other people.

Laws of the Ninja

There are four rules that the Ninja prepares for combat. These laws grant the Ninja the liberty to do what is needed to take on their foe.

ANONYMITY

The Ninja should always remain his intentions and thoughts from his adversaries. This is essential when planning a Ninja's mission. Even those who are close to the Ninja do not have access to the details of the mission. The less people who are aware of anything, the more knowledgeable.

EXPLOITATION

The Ninja has to make use of everything and everything in order to beat his adversaries. To achieve this to do this, the Ninja examines each aspect that affects his adversaries presence. The aim of this data gathering is to identify and exploit every way.

TRICKERY

The Ninja must keep his adversaries in a state of confusion as to what is actually happening and what is illusion. By doing this, the opponent is never sure what to expect. when they aren't sure of what is expected, they are unable to make a plan for defending.

Strategy

The Ninja never reacts by relying on random emotions. Strategizing is the key to success. The Ninja must come up with a variety of strategies for action and each plan should include a contingency plan. Then, not only should the Ninja succeed, they must be stylish in their victory.

THE NINJA'S DOCTRINES

There are many practices taught in those of the Kurai Kotori family. The teachings of the clan have been handed through generations of families in several of Japan's Martial Traditions.

MICHI

Michi means the "Path." It is the path followed by Ninja is to develop the mind, body and soul throughout their life. The process is frequently described as "Musha Shugyo" also known as "Warrior Cultivation." Even even though it sounds like a mystery, there isn't way to fail when it comes to achieving. The past was when Musha Shugyo could be achieved through traveling to various Bujutsu school and challenging the best student to battle. In this way, the Ninja faced the most brutal form of combat in which they either triumphed or died. While this type of thing seems like a flimsy idea however the idea behind it is quite innovative. In the most intense of situations, you'll surely gain increased awareness during combat. The acute sense Ninja acquired through Musha Shugyo helped them combat the enemy as swiftly as possible, not risking anything that could alter their abilities to prevail.

Shugyo

The Kurai Kotori Ryu, the concept of Musha Shugyo is an important aspect of the Ninja's training. It helps the Ninja to maximize the benefits of any situation by never taking everything as a given. Every combat scenario, the Ninja must have "Seishi of Choetsu" that is,"Seishi O Choetsu" or "Transcending thoughts of life and death" aware that they must cherish every moment of their life, so that when they die they will depart from the physical world knowing that they utilized all the opportunities in their lives to the maximum capacity.

Life and death

NAKA-IMA

To be a powerful person To remain powerful, the Ninja need to constantly increase their understanding. It is only the way for them to live an abundant life. Old and new complement one another, but they remain distinct entities. One way of join them into one entity is to see everything as an integral part of the "Eternal today," that is, the "Forever present" idea. This notion dictates that combat arts are developed by focusing on the exponents of earlier times as well as the current knowledge that is available in the present. It is understood to be aware that, if the craft wants to develop, the modern cannot ever replace the older.

Perseverance

NIN

The notion that is "Nin" is frequently described as "Perseverance" or "Strength," but what is really at stake is "Mental Attitude." This mental attitude is what distinguishes those who are Ninja from the common Martial artist. The Ninja's mental state can be manifested in their goals for themselves. To become an expert in unarmed combat is just one of their objectives They also need to achieve proficiency with any weapon, and become skilled in making elixirs, poisons and explosives, be able to remain undetected in disguise, achieve elegance in climbing the highest peaks, stealth, and acrobatics and be proficient in the art of survival, concealment, and infiltration techniques. These are only some of the goals for Ninjas, in addition to countless other. The main thing that it all boils to is growth. Anything that will provide the Ninja insights into themselves can be considered an aspect of the Kurai Kotori Tradition.

SHIBUMI

When the Ninja is proficient in a variety of subjects, they reach the state of "Shibumi," which is often known in the sense of "Simplicity" of both the body and the mind. When Shibumi takes effect and the Ninja is a graceful and elegant warrior that makes even the most complicated of tasks appear as an easy task that requires only a little thought.

KI

Ki represents Ki is the "Energy" that is found in every living thing. It is not visible or touched, it just exists. Ki is apparent when the body and mind work in perfect harmony. Although the process of developing Ki isn't an easy process but it is necessary when one wants to harness the full potential of one's self.

The first thing a Ninja should be focusing on is the correct practice of physical techniques since when the body is balanced and controlled, Ninja's Ki will start to grow. Training in physical form must be completed before mental development will be achieved. A lot of Ninja are so consumed by the notion of developing a powerful power that they are obsessed with the thought. They are eager to skip the physical training to learn the secret chanting that can open the door to the ultimate power. The power of this kind is only accessible to those who develop their energy in a steady and persistently.

The same technique of self-concentration that is used to teach the Ninja physically can be applied at the beginning of developing the mind. The key is awareness. of concentration, and learning to see the smallest aspects in everything. Through the Ninja's training in mentality, it is essential to become aware of such arts as calligraphy carpentry, painting, pottery and theater, as through these forms of expression, the Ninja learns to master the art of focus and dedication to the highest level of quality of detail.

Hara

Ki flows throughout in the "Hara," or "Stomach region." It can be considered the most potent part within the body of a Ninja, because it is the home of the center of Ki in the deepest part of the body. This area inside is referred to as "Seika no itten" also known as the "Vital spot," and it is thought to be the point the place where the body and the mind join, resulting in the most powerful expression of energy that is balanced within the body. Hara is the term used to describe the Hara is employed to help the Ninja lets all their life energy to fall to their core point. Once this is achieved the body and mind become one, which allows the Ninja's power to be focused and controlled.

KIAI

Kiai is translated as "Intense energy" and is frequently taken to mean a simple yell at the Ninja during an attack. Yet, Kiai houses a much more profound significance. Kiai could be described as an emotion that is raw, like an expression of the spirit that a Ninja unleashes onto the physical world. Many art forms stress Kiai due to the fact that it requires people to breathe while they are execution of the techniques, however, this isn't the whole capabilities of Kiai.

There are certain sound effects that are released according to the action is taken by the Ninja. In the event that the Ninja is fighting with their Kiai is a loud scream that comes out of their Hara and makes a sort sound that resembles the "Ei" noise. If the Ninja's strike is successful, their Kiai transforms to "Ei-yah," which signifies "Zanshin," or "Remaining spirit" following a skillful technique. If the Ninja is thrown or struck the Ninja should release an accepting Kiai which makes the sound "Toh," which armors their body to absorb the impact. But this is not the whole amount of Kiai. There is a Kurai Kotori clan also has Kiai that is a Kiai that doesn't make any sound. It's known as a hidden shout and is used to concentrate the energy of one's. True Kiai is recognized by someone who has practiced their art for a long time. It's the vibe that they give off, a feeling that makes them stand out from the rest. They are able to grab your attention with every move.

AIKI

Aiki can be described as "Internal energy" and is a symbol of harmony inside the Ninja. The energy emanates out of the Ninja who radiates an unwavering and calm spirit that is able to penetrate an enemy's mindand destroy the desire to fight.

The achievement of Aiki is not a requirement it just occurs. It is, in essence, Aiki is the process of overcoming the enemy using only the mind, and just a glance is all that's required to completely defeat anyone who blocks the path of the Ninja's aim.

IN and YO

The idea that of In the concept of In and Yo (yin and Yang) is an integral part in the Ninja's method of living. It is because in its depths, the Ninja is able to realize that there is a complete equilibrium between the negative and positive forces that make up the universe. In attaining this knowledge, the Ninja is able to see the world as a wholeand realize the fact that In and Yo are equally important to the scheme of things.

Being aware that good and evil or right and wrong and darkness and light are two perspectives on the same thing makes the Ninja the advantage. They realize that there only balance and imbalance. The Ninja must work in harmony to In as well as Yo to fix any weaknesses inside its structure. This means that when one is stronger than the other , the Ninja must recognize the difference and work to rectify it.

The balance is evident within the internal processes of nature. The sun and moon always perform the same task of rising , setting and rising again, providing us both darkness and light without thinking about it. If the sun was to become predominant over the moon the planetary system would change and life in the way we see it today would be gone forever. Although this may be an example of a large scale balance, it's similar in all aspects. It doesn't matter how easy it appears... equilibrium has to be maintained.

In and Yo

In the event of applying In or Yo to fight, it must be noted that the balance rests with the participants. What determines who is the winner and the loser isn't determined by the fact that someone is correct or not or who is either good or evil, since these variables have no impact on the outcomes of a fight. Battle success is dependent on the ability and plan. Do not misinterpret this fact.

Chapter 11: Philosophical Foundations

To tap into the true essence of a warrior, clan members from the Kurai Kotori clan are instructed to imagine the entirety of their training experiences as occurring within the vastness of a spiritual forest. To enhance this vision members of the clan see themselves as one of the numerous creatures living within the the forest. In keeping this mental image that way, the Ninja will realize that they are element of nature, one part of a larger puzzle. The importance of the forest mindset is apparent when one considers the forest's residents. There are many species that live within the boundaries of the forest. Each animal is distinct. Like each Ninja. The individuality of each Ninja is the key to the forest. Without diversity it would be impossible to have conflict. And without conflict one would not have the requirement to be a warrior. However, a world without conflict is not a natural thing. For as long as mankind was around, there has been wars in all forms, from massive battles between nations and civil wars to arguments between people. The motives behind these battles are not relevant. The lesson isn't. You must remember that in all things, you will encounter opposition.

"The Forest of Insight

The same opposition exists in nature, too. But the Ninja who lives in the forest of the spirit tries to accept the idea of conflict. Every creature of the forest is believed as natural enemies. It is a fact. Even animals that do not pose a apparent threat to other creatures are the most likely targets for adversaries. Simply because a animal is passive by nature does not mean that those that surround him are following the same lifestyle. For instance that the fact that the wild deer is living in a manner that presents no danger to other animals of the forest doesn't suggest that the mountain lion which is following him may think twice about eating him. It's all about instinct. Hunter, and one who hunts. Each is talented in different zones. The mountain lion can be armed with strength and cunning and the deer is a beast of quickness and agility. The key to victory is that one both have a greater awareness of their surroundings. This is the same principle that determines the survival of a Ninja in the forest of spirituality. It's not about being faster or stronger but an issue of who is more conscious. Therefore it is important that a Ninja shouldn't feel like they need to be hunter to stay alive.

They should simply improve their sense of danger and then react to it.

The Natural Law of Nature

Nature supplies the Ninja with the necessary raw ingredients needed to develop themselves to the best of their ability. The forest is home to all the elements of nature that act as the Ninja's instructors. Water, earth, and wind. They are all in complete harmony in the forest. The Ninja's mission is to discover this harmony within the elements.

Four Primary Elements Four Primary Elements

THE POOL of knowledge

In the deepest reaches of the forest, there is a tranquil swimming pool that even though it is small it reveals a deep. This pool represents the infinite amount of knowledge available to those who seek more understanding. The pool is where all the creatures of the forest meet to satisfy curiosity. The pool, in reality, can be described as an actual Dojo as is the woods all which surrounds it. The Ninja is attracted to the pool, not just to drink the life-giving nourishment it provides but also to look at their reflections as they expand with every drink. This is sole spot in the forest where all animals share. It is a spot of gathering in which all animals come together.

A Reflection Space

THE POWER WITHIN

In every Ninja there is an untapped power waiting to come out. It is the force spiritual that each Ninja will base their learning. The process of emergence of the Ninja's powers are not a quick process however. Like everything good take time. For the Ninja this power is as an animal totem referred to as"Bugo, "Bugo," or "Martial Name." These are far greater than the overly dramatic names that are given to the Ninja to promote creating ego-poisoning. The Ninja gets this name from the Jonin after they have proved they are worthy of this honour. When the Ninja's identity has been made public, they are entitled to having the image engraved on their right shoulder or arm by means of the aid of an Irezumi (tattoo). The significance of the tattoo is its effect on the warrior wearing the design. The tattoo acts as an aesthetic reminder to Ninjas Ninja that they are unique, as well as serving as a focus point to help them develop their fighting abilities.

THE INTERNATIONAL FORGE

The possibilities of adventure when submerged in the forest's depths is limitless. Adventure is where you will find it. It is only by spotting opportunities as they arise will the Ninja be successful. Adventure is a synonym for "Challenge," but its meaning is quite evident. You must be able to experience all emotions including anger, fear happiness, anger, sadness, despair, love and confusion. These emotions are all present in the forest and it's the way the Ninja manages the emotions that are important. Adventure is a method of applying, it's taking the knowledge and wisdom of the water and applying it for direct experiences. This is where one can discover wisdom. It isn't the only result of getting older. Actually it is a quality that is acquired through overcoming obstacles and utilizing the knowledge gained to develop maturity in judgement. To develop the ability to grow However, one must first take the step to tackle the obstacles they face. This is why we have"the "Internal Forge." The forge is a part of the subconscious of the Ninja, and is the process of overcoming doubt. If a problem arises it is the Ninja should be ready to face the fires of the forge, so that they are tempered by the experiences. Going to the forge is a way of discovering the mental, physical and spiritual value in oneself. For the individual Ninja this test of the spirit can last for several hours. Some are attuned to their inner fires in a flash, while others take their time. But, time doesn't matter and ultimately, we have to confront ourselves.

The fire in

The Law of the Wild

The survival in the forest is extremely difficult. There is no easy way to survive. While the forest offers plenty of security, the forest also poses dangers. Be aware that the forest is not enemy or friend However, it has the capacity to house both. An Ninja who is in the wilderness has to remain vigilant, aware that the ally of today could turn into tomorrow's foe. This is the rule of nature. This is a valid philosophies due to the fact that everyone has the right to follow their own moral standards. A person might not agree with an individual's way of living however, conflict usually comes without consequence. One should not be able to judge the way of life of the other. This is evident in a small portion of my personal philosophical stance. This philosophy states "I was not put here on earth to conform to the morals of other people. My purpose is to challenge the thinking of warriors that are yet to become. My training methods are often extreme, however, I'll never let go of trying to realize the goals that are buried within the minds of those following me. I'm the epitome of neutrality and can do anything at any moment." I believe it is due to this understanding of me that I'm competent in strengthening my students. I will do whatever needs to be done to improve their capabilities. I accomplish this by having them go through a variety of stressful situations to test their mental and physical endurance. Keep in mind that you have two sides of each coin. If you're competent to stand up during positive times, and then falter in times that seem unfavorable circumstances, you're only half an ace. I just hope that in the course of the course of their lives that everyone will discover them in this manner, to not be compelled to criticize other people. When one is able to accept the person they are as then they'll be able recognize their role in the larger view of life. When this happens, one recognizes the flaw in being a judge of another because they don't follow the same set of rules. It doesn't matter how you feel or what you say that everyone has to live according to their own standards.

This kind of thinking is a process that takes time to develop in the realm of the Ninja. It is essential that they avoid the error of viewing other people in the shadow of their own shortcomings. Only when the Ninja suffers the same infringement, and focuses on their own ideals, will an necessary light shine through to erase the shadow within their own eyes. In this instance, the saying "Be cautious about judging others in case you want to be judged" is of great significance.

One Warrior, One Art

The Ninja must have complete faith that they are learning the correct system to learn. Through the years, I've seen a lot of students come at me with concerns that the previous martial art they learned did not cover all types of fighting. They would complain that they were never given the chance to engage in ground combat while others were astonished at the fact that they had not learned weapons, and so on. The point is that they believed that something was lacking. While I'm proud of the fact that my teaching methods are diverse I am also sad that my students are quick to point out the flaws in other methods. Many arts are focused on particular aspects of fighting, but their most serious flaw is passing judgement on them too early. Each art is taught to students a particular method to deal with their opponents. In Karate the focus is on power and raw strength. In Aikido the emphasis is on redirecting energy. When it comes to Jujutsu students are taught how to manage and to immobilize. Although this is only an illustration, what it demonstrates is that every martial art is unique and has its distinct strategy for combat. A lot of students see these distinct methods as weak and try to rectify the issue by combining training in different disciplines in hopes of gaining more techniques. I am not a fan of this strategy. My experience has shown that the methods and the principles used by different styles tend to clash which makes it difficult to integrate them into a coherent fighting system. I believe that a student must be thoughtful before deciding on their option, and, once they have decided the path, they should be as faithful as priests. In the end, any art has the potential to be successful but the individual who practices it must remain committed long enough to discover its secrets. Keep in mind, "One warrior, one art." Do not confuse yourself.

Learn the principles of your art by observing discipline. At the end, you will be blessed.

STAYING FIXED

The mind needs to be prevented from wandering, as it is incredibly easily to wander off from the track. At one point, we are certain of our goal, and then we begin to question the very existence of us. That's the nature of our existence. That's why the Ninja should be strong in the face of anything that could disrupt their training. If there is one thing that is certain it is that lots of situations will come up to hinder. These challenges have been set for the Ninja and should they surrender in...they have admitted defeat. What it boils to is motivation. While the teacher's role is to guide them on their way, it's up on the student to find motivation to learn. Students must be aware that what they put into their path is what they'll receive from it. The most important objective for each student should be to remain focussed on a goal. This objective is to collect details from the teacher and take in it, absorb it, and then perfect it.

The purpose of training

A lot of people who take on the road of the warrior will ask them this query. "Why should I train?" This is a question that can have multiple answers. But, I think the training of a student is determined by their own individual preparation for life and the obstacles that they might encounter during their journey. There shouldn't be a one focal aspect. Self-protection, weaponry, strategy, survival, stealth, mysticism. These skills are vital to be able to adjust to any situation as they happen. This makes finding the most precise reason to be able to do so because it is impossible to know for certain what the future will bring. This is why being without an unrealized goal. This is essential because when one is training for a specific motive, they may confine themselves to a single purpose. If one's mind is open and willing to change, their learning will continue to evolve and adapt and make the art it is to study the instrument utilized to attain more understanding.

SIMPLE PHILOSOPHY

Since I started teaching the art of the Ninja back in the 1980s, there's been one particular question that has been asked by nearly every student. This one is what kind of belief system or philosophy is this Kurai Kotori Ninja live by? This is a difficult issue that has a variety of answers. I'll try my best to clarify.

In the first place, the Kurai Kotori Ninja should develop their skills in a constructive way. This can only be achieved by utilizing the experiences of their lives to learn how they can be more effective with situations that happen in their lives. What I am trying to convey is there exist a lot of dangers in our lives that are unavoidable. It is possible to try to avoid them but eventually they will be able to catch up with us. We could take those experiences in the aim of whether or not taking the result positively which encourages the growth. We'll make friends and enemies. We will be able to find affection and hate. We will fight and love peace. We will achieve successes, but also be stricken by losses. We will live, and we will end up dying. All of these and more will occur as we travel through the world. What is important are our choices when travelling. The meaning behind the message I'm trying to convey lies within each of us. Our choices made in every moment of lives influence the people who surround us. The only advice I have to offer is "Make an impact." Don't just sit at the unfolding of events and become part of the events.

There are many who are quick highlight all the flaws in the world. Hunger, crime, and corruption. They are real. exist, but I've got some insight to share with you. It is much more easy to accept your preconceptions and avoid making changes. It's hard to be respectful, to listen, to speak and accept the lessons you learn could alter your life. When you live this way, students can overcome discrimination based on race, gender, or any other mind-altering conviction and instead live life in a positive way.

Do not mislead yourself in any way about what I'm telling you. I am in no way suggesting how one should live their lives. I'm simply saying that everyone should be aware of the events that happen in their lives. The decisions they make in their lives is theirs to make.

Multiple paths, one destination

Every person who learns an art of combat is embarking on a individual quest that has to be respect. There are many different ways to practice the same style , and people do not adhere to the same faith. It is important to remember that the Kurai Kotori Ninja should always express gratitude to those who practice martial arts regardless of their style or affiliation. Remember that it's not the way to practice it but the person who is studying it. If they're devoted students who are committed to their studies then that's enough. There are others who you meet along the way that are loud and arrogant who claim to be unbeatable, their manner of speaking is the best or some other insanity-filled rant. They should be avoided since the only thing they're doing is creating an imbalanced energy and, consequently, bad luck. If you are unable to avoid them, or if they are not an option, then do the things you need to.

Chapter 12: Physical Preparation

Five physical skills are necessary to be an efficient Ninja. Flexibility, Strength, Endurance, Balance and agility. The body requires rigorous training to improve the efficacy of these characteristics.

Strength PRACTICES

The development of physical strength to enhance the ability of a person to apply and withstand the force. Training for strength should be considered a complement, not a hinderance. That means one must not boost muscles at the expense of speed or flexibility. However, strong and healthy muscles can generate explosive strength that's the type of strength that is sought by Ninjas. Ninja.

MAKIWARA

One of the most neglected aspects of training for strength is makiwara daily practice. Makiwara refer to "Striking targets" that are used to train the feet and hands to do maximum damage. Makiwara can come in a variety of shapes. A wood plank that is that is buried beneath the ground with its top part covered with thin padding, a wall-mounted target that is covered with canvas and padding or even a large trunk of wood , with small padded targets placed on the surface.

Makiwara Design

STRIKING THE MAKIWARA

The primary method used in makiwara conditioning is to use the tightening of the fist (striking with the two topmost knuckles) as well as the toe strike (striking using the foot's ball). Both of these are among the strongest body weapons employed to attack with thrusts. But, other body weapons (elbows knees, knees, and head) can be trained through hitting the makiwara boards. Regular practice has produced punches that have a weight of close to 2000 pounds. per square inch. This is the highest could be. A long-term sequence of repeated exercises prepares the muscles of the body to absorb the impact of an injury. It builds strength, strength and Kime (focused power). In order to be an Ninja it is required to strike the makiwara at least 50 times in a single hand, each training session. This helps the student to be fully committed to every hit.

MUSHIN

Makiwara training also helps to develop Mushin, which is often translated as "no thinking." "Mu" meaning negation, "Shin" meaning heart, mind, feeling. "No mind" is an Zen phrase that refers to the condition of mind clarity as well as improved sense (sensory as well as intuitive) often referred to in the context of "pure mental state," produced by the absence of conscious thoughts or judgments, thoughts or emotions (fear or anxiety) and preconception or self-consciousness. For the Ninja practicing the practice of meditation (towards the mushin) is an essential complement to training in technical aspects. Mushin allows the mind to be not inactive, it's completely free. Not impeded, slowed or distracted The mind has the freedom to comprehend, respond, and take action. The mind isn't fixed on anything , but is free to be open to all things; it is expanded throughout the entire body, with complete attention to and awareness of all things.

The Makiwara

HORIZONTAL POLE

A horizontal pole can be a must for strength training in Ninjas and there's a range of exercises that utilize poles of various sizes.

HANGING

The first and most important thing is that the Ninja can be hung by the hands while palms are facing towards the front to stretch shoulders and arms. To make it more challenging tiny bags of sand may be placed on shoulders similar to saddlebags. The aim is to hang for as long as you can, without touching your heels to the floor. It is possible to hang the Ninja is also able to hang upside-down by folding legs in over the pole, allow your body to swing by extending the arms. While this is a strength exercise, it's also an effective endurance exercise.

Affixed to a Horizontal Pole

PULLL UPS

The pull-ups are performed by putting your palms inwards and outwards as well as using two hands or single hands. This is a great exercise for shoulders, arms, and the back muscle. It can also be done by putting small rope loops onto the pole where wrists could be placed into and allowing the biceps muscles to get the most attention.

Pull-ups on a Horizontal Pole

DIPS

The upward movement of lifting off posts that are vertical is extremely efficient for strengthening the chest and triceps.

The dips in between two objects

ELEVATED PRASH UPS

Push ups that are performed by putting your feet on an elevated object will allow the Ninja to increase the effectiveness of a typical push-up. This exercises the chest and the shoulders and the triceps. To intensify the workout the Ninja can do the push up using the finger tips or fore knuckles to build their strike weapons. The most challenging form of the workout is to do it using the ridge hand, with the arms spread out further.

The push-ups are elevated on an object

Receiving the IMPACTS

Physical strength in the face of a strike is as crucial as, if not more as delivering a strong strike. In combat fighting, the Ninja is required to close the distance in order to strike, and, in doing so, get into the striking distance of their adversaries. This is the crucial range the place where counterattacks and attacks be swiftly moving at a rapid speed...and in this situation, the chance of being hit is nearly certain. So, the limbs as well as the torso need to be trained to withstand these hits. This can be accomplished in through a variety of methods.

BAMBOO SWORD

It is the first thing to do is take repeatedly striking the forearms and shins with the Chikuto (bamboo sword). The strikes do not need to be fully forceful but they must provide an enormous amount of energy to strengthen the body's natural defenses.

Incorporating the slash of the bamboo sword

ABSORBING KICKS

The legs and the torso must be strengthened through receiving thrusting and circular kicks. The focus should be on the ability to adapt the posture of the body in order to absorb the energy from the bigger muscles. While physical strength is essential but it must be remembered that breathing properly is essential in the event of a blow since even though the body is strained the air must be able to circulate freely to maintain a certain amount of flexibility to help disperse the energy incoming.

Incorporating strikes to the body

ENDURANCE Drills

Endurance drills are designed to enhance the Ninja's capacity to endure physical stress for prolonged period of time. Physical endurance can be improved by performing specific exercises and the correct breathing techniques.

STRADDLE LEG POSITION

Leg strength and flexibility are important within the hips. This is the most significant overall. It is important to be flexible in all aspects. Ninja could be required to climb, remain low in order to move, or stay hidden for an extended amount of duration. It is crucial to keep the thighs horizontal and the back straight throughout this workout since dropping too low in the straddle will negate the beneficial effects.

Straddle leg position

CLAY POTS

The arms extended out to towards the sides while gripping an opening in a clay-based pot puts pressure on arms and legs while simultaneously improving the grip strength. The pots are filled with different quantities of clay or sand in order to raise the weight to meet the requirements of the particular Ninja that is using the pots. The objective of the workout is to keep the pots in place as long as is possible without dropping your arms or making the grip weak. The exercise can be done with the straddle position to increase the level of difficulty. Beyond the initial stage, the kettles may be extended to the side or turned to the side to alter the energy distribution and put pressure on various muscles of the forearms and shoulders.

Clay pots that grip.

WRINGING CLOTH

To increase forearm endurance and twisting strength , the Ninja utilizes a large piece of cloth that is soaked in water. The force of counter twisting is applied to the cloth in order to squeeze away the liquid. The cloth is then twisted until there is no water left. It is immersed in water and the process is repeated.

Water dripping from an untidy cloth

JUMP LUNGES

The hip and leg muscles require a the most intense of workouts which can be done by jumping lunges.

Alternating Jump Lunges

FLEXIBILITY Drills

When the notion of flexibility is mentioned initially, one's thoughts are generally about leg fractures. But, the concept of stretching is about increasing the body's flexibility when it is bent, turned, or bent. This means that each joint and bend within the body must be trained to the point that they are more flexible and less susceptible to injuries.

SHOULDERS

Shoulder stretches can be performed using the hands of the opposite shoulder, while pulling the left elbow to the left. This exercise must be performed with both hands and then performed in small circular rotations using both shoulders.

Shoulder flexibility

WRISTS

The wrists need to be stretched out by putting hands palms on palms, ensuring they are together as you apply downward pressure on the towards the front. Then, the wrists must be stretched outward, with the palms facing outward while applying pressure on the back of the hand using the other hand.

Flexible wrist

BACK

Stretching the back out by lying face down and expanding the torso by extending the arms , while making sure that the hips are flat against the floor. When you are seated the right leg is stretched to the outside, while the left leg is pulled back and placed over your right knee. The right arm is then placed to the right side of the knee, as the left arm is twisted towards the rear.

Back flexibility

HIPS

Begin in a lunge with the left leg in front and the left arm put under the left knee and focusing upon pushing your chest towards the ground. A seated position with the feet positioned together is taken. Your feet will be pulled forward by the hands, while the elbows apply downward pressure on the legs.

Hip flexibility

LEGS

A side lunge is performed by extending the left leg and the other leg on its side, bending below the body. The pressure is applied subtly by leaning back into the stretch. The position is then alternated. Then, one foot is placed into the loop of a rope that is linked to the pulley. The rope is pulled using hands to ensure that the foot is at an easy stretch.

Leg flexibility

BALANCE Drills

Ability to change in a particular location without losing control and falling.

HANDSTAND BALANCE

They are placed hands on the floor and the feet are extended upwards with an occasional bend at the knees.

Balance on the hands

PILLAR BALANCE

Balanced on one foot and standing on an object for 10 counts. After the timer, legs switch by jumping up and down, while switching the foot positions.

Balancing on one pillar

BALANCE ON BEAM

Moving forward and backward on a beam that is horizontal will increase the centerline balance. To increase the difficulty you can leap up and then turn the body into the air, and then fall back on the beam in towards the reverse direction.

Balancing on beams

AGILITY DRUGS

Agility is the ability of Ninjas to slam on the brakes, alter direction, and accelerate once more.

SLOOPING WALL

A steeply angled wall will enhance one's ability to modify the body's weight and speed.

The surface can be angled to the point of running up

LEAPING AROUND

Jumping up on something will enhance the capacity to measure the amount of force required to propel the body in the air and to land on a platform that is raised. It is also extremely effective for endurance exercises.

The act of jumping onto an elevated object

STRAIGHTENING DOWNWARD

A leap that descends is about jumping up and outward simultaneously so that the body falls straight down, rather than being angular. The energy of landing needs to be evenly distributed between the knees, hips and ankles. The landing may be made straight into a roll to more evenly distribute energy.

The jump off of an elevated object

AVOIDING PROJECTILES

The ability to intuitively and precisely propel your body in a specific direction is essential. Beware of projectiles that are thrown at you. ability by assessing the direction of the object with a single notice , and avoid its impact.

Beware of objects that are thrown

Endless Alternatives

There are numerous exercises that go beyond the ones within this guide. It is crucial that the Ninja keep their focus on the continuous growth the body's temple. The exact exercises may change however the result is the same.

Chapter 13: Historical Ties

They Ninja in Japan are among the most famous spy agents that in the history of mankind. But, the phrase "Ninja" is a reference to a variety of people who operated within and outside of the rules that governed the Japanese Feudal government. The "Ninja" came from all kinds of classes of people.

Ninja Hero

Ninja Mystic

It is impossible to know the motives and adventures of these warriors as their true origins are obscure. There was not a single person who was the originator of the methods and philosophies which comprised the practice that has now been referred to as "Ninjutsu" (the practice of persistence and stealth). In reality, much of what we know regarding the Ninja is usually exaggerated and interpreted as legend and myth. According to the historian of the day, the Ninja was either a hero, vagabond, mystic, terrorist or assassin or tradesman. Any of these assertions could be true. Anyone who has enough motivation and skills could be able to follow the path of the shadow warrior. The term "ninja" can refer to anyone. Ninja can be anybody and even Buddhist priests were not shy of taking the cloak and dagger method to protect their temples from untrustworthy pirates. One thing historians all agree on was that Ninja's commitment to the method of deceit and intrigue was unmatched.

It is now my turn to play the role of historian. Through my many years of studying the Japanese martial arts, I've been exposed to an immense amount of information. In order to pay tribute to the warriors referred to as Ninja I'm going to provide an abbreviated account of crucial events that led to the creation and development of the art of Ninjutsu. While it is my responsibility as historian "interpret" the historical past, it's also my responsibility to view it from different angles and, often, results in the creation of an "reinterpreted" the past. This is crucial since many historians view subjects from a singular viewpoint. They create a narrative that is most appropriate to their perspective. In many instances, writers from Japanese culture approach their work from a particularly gruesome perspective that Ninja are portrayed as black-clad villains that murder their victims without guilt or regrets. This is truly tragic. It's like saying that every cowboy from the

American West was a gunfighter who had no respect for law and law and. This isn't the case. It is crucial to be aware that every single person born has their own unique mind. Human beings aren't robots that just wander around as zombies doing pre-programmed tasks. Humans are a factor that is indisputable. While it is more easy to see the entire race, class or even a culture as one way or another but it's also a bit ignorant. It is necessary to remove the blinders for a while to examine all the possibilities, and realize that, no matter how much we believe we are certain ....we were not there. This is the reason I have always sought to free my learners from rigidity of facts in order to develop a greater knowledge of Ninja. But, there are certain historical events that cannot be debated. The time wars were fought in the past, who lived and passed away, and many other events were documented in great detail by historians of the day. We can only hope that these scribes from feudal times were honest and tried to write an accurate record of events instead of being driven by politics to write about things that would make the person they were serving look nice in the eyes of the following generations. We'll just have to hope that this was the situation.

Ninja Scrolls

Although we can learn much from these records but what happened to the information that wasn't recorded? We are only able to speculate about the various deeds executed in the many thousands of Ninja that lived through the history of Japan. The scrolls and the books that exist are where the majority of historians collect what data they are able to. They only cover a tiny amount of what happened over the various generations. Even though these documents have proven very useful in helping create a clear picture of the activities Ninja was up to, the reality is that the vast majority of Ninja activities were probably not noticed and that's logical. Only those missions with a very notable would be extensively recorded due to the huge impact their actions had across the entire country. It is likely, if not immediately apparent there was a chance that Ninja also carried out hundreds of smaller-scale operations which had more subtle impacts on the people surrounding them. There are numerous instances in which Ninja were the ones responsible for stopping conflicts before they started and where a few pieces of information were collected to establish alliances, certain undesirables that could have caused trouble were removed and when an adversary's weaknesses were identified to ensure swift victory if war had to be fought. If these were not the more subtle missions, there are a lot of historical events that could have been dramatically changed. But, since my speculation is not relevant, and we should start our search with the historical record.

CHINESE IMPULSION

From the writings that have a place, it's apparent that the underlying ideas that would eventually evolve into Ninjutsu were derived from China. The source of this information is the Chinese text about the Military arts , also known in the book "The The Art of War" which was composed by the famous strategist Sun Tzu (400-320 B.C.). The extensive knowledge in the writings of Sun Tzu contained details on tactical maneuvering and the psychology of war selecting objectives with care as well as how to plan an appropriate offensive, the importance of surprise, necessity for a united command and the most important thing, keeping the secrecy of. This knowledge was first introduced to Japan in the sixth century. In the years following that time the skills of strategic thinking were developed and developed by a group of mystic shamans, known by the name of "Yamabushi," which roughly means "One who rests at night in mountains."

Yamabushi

These warrior-mystics are thought to be the forerunners to the Ninja. They practiced the martial arts of Shugendo that were a combination from Buddhism, Shinto, Taoism as well as Folklore. Priests also had training on their Chinese martial arts that many would agree that was the foundation for the development of many of the combat skills that were unarmed and weaponry techniques that were developed in Japan.

CREATURES OF HEROIC

It was also at this period that stories about "Karasu tengu" which is also known as "Crow goblins" came to light. The creatures were believed to possess the human body as well as the wings and head of birds. They were believed to have magic powers like the ability to teleport and spell casting. Karasu tengu were believed to be a bit sly in their behavior, afflicting all who passed through their territory with a myriad different tricks, traps and tricks.

Karasu tengu

Karasu Tengu were believed to be formidable warriors who had the highest level of skill in combat, specifically when it came to swordsmanship. They interacted with each other via telepathy, rather than through using the written word. There was also a claim that they had the ability to communicate with humans, and could project themselves into the dream world of warriors to share special knowledge, like unique techniques for fighting or spiritual wisdom. Rarely they could also change into human forms to interact with humans. The warriors of the greatest skill were believed to have killed and fought an opponent known as a Karasu Tengu, however they were shocked when their adversary would transform to a wounded bird right before their sight.

Though these stories were more myth than fact and were a bit skewed, it was a fascinating coincident the Tengu and Yamabushi were also believed to have mystical powers similar to those that were derived from practices that were practiced in mountain sanctuary. As time passed, legends about Yamabushi as well as Tengu were interspersed. A new type of Tengu came into existence.

Yamabushi-Tengu

They were referred to in the form of "Yamabushi-tengu," or "Mountain goblins." They were Tengu had more humanity than the previous. Yamabushi Tengu were believed to be elderly men with bare feet sporting long noses, and hair of white. The long-nosed human-tengu were generally responsible for bird-tengu. The most powerful of Tengu was named Sojobo and was known for teaching Minamoto Yoshitsune secret of Kurama Hachi-ryu Yamabushi in the Kurama Hachi-ryu Yamabushi temple located on Mount Kurama.

Sojobo instructs Minamoto Yoshitsune

In the following decades in Japan The stories of Tengu were popular and their connection to the people who would later become popularly referred to as "Ninja," was inevitable. Like every culture, tales of myth and legends always have a basis in reality. The imagination is a link to reality. Today these things are regarded as a fable, but in the past the ability to think creatively of the mind allowed people to achieve extraordinary feats. So, having a conviction in something can make it true.

SPIRITUAL SWORD WARRIORS

In the 6th century, numerous Buddhist monks arrived from China to establish Temples throughout Japan. A lot of Japanese considered this to be an attempt to undermine the well-established Shinto religion. It was inevitable that conflict would arise. So, the monks cultivated an combat system known as "Chuan Fa" that was derived from the martial arts that were learned by the Shaolin of China.

Shaolin Monk

In Japan the art was called "Kempo." In the beginning, the only weapon employed by monks was their staff, however, to protect their religion they also began to be renowned with spears, halberds, and the axe. The priests who learned these techniques were referred to in the form of "Sohei,"or "Warrior-monks." As time, because of the constant changes in the religion, it became imperative for these monks come up with a different system called "Himitsu Kempo" which translates to "Secret fist of the law." The art form was developed as an effective method of fighting in the dark and not using fists. The Sohei utilized information gathering to help achieve their mission of gaining the true freedom of religion.

Sohei Warrior

Even though these monks became adept at spying but there were things they couldn't perform due to their vows of faith. Due to these limitations they Sohei were able to turn to the people who resided in the nearby villages. A lot of them relied on temples for wisdom and direction. The Sohei taught a lot of the commoners Shaolin Monks in both the martial and religious arts. A few of these women and men were later referred to in the form of "Jisamurai," or "Rural warriors," many of whom were foot soldiers for the warlords in the provinces where they lived. Some of these rural warriors were trained in the techniques of Himitsu Kempo in order to aid the monks in their espionage activities. A lot of the specially trained warriors were extremely committed to the religious aspects of their training and performed their espionage duties in way to demonstrate their faith. The skills they were taught by the warriors later evolved to "Nimpo," or the "Law of patience." Since patience is among the top prominent virtues found in any religion It was their dedication to this notion that allowed them to be so successful. A Nimpo warrior would not make rash decisions, but rather rely on gathering information as well as strategic thinking to guarantee victory. They would also avoid engaging with adversaries in battle. Due to their subversive actions and their subversive activities, the Buddhist temples would later become an extremely influential and powerful organizations in Japan. Outside of their role as Nimpo warriors, other groups tried to utilize the expertise from the Sohei to defend their villages from bandsits, defend themselves from marauding army and to lead rebellions against the unfair taxation forced on them from the state. In contrast to their religious affiliations the tactics employed by these women and men were primarily focused on deceit using techniques such as surprise attack assassination, poisoning, fraud and destruction. The art of Ninjutsu was beginning to develop.

The first organized NINJA Groups

The real roots for the first Ninja appear to be rooted in two areas in the Suzuka mountain range, in which there were two mountain ranges: Yamabushi as well as the Sohei were believed to have been located. These regions were referred to by the names of Iga (ee-ga) as well as Koga (koo-ga). They were extremely closely related to one another culturally as well as politically. Koga was actually region from the Omi province, and Iga was a distinct region its own, however in all aspects, the two regions were expected to constitute part of the same region. In the Suzuka mountains were a mystery composed of a dense terrain, which made traveling extremely difficult. Due to this, it became a refuge for traitors, renegades and thieves with no other choice.

Iga/Koga Region

In the Heian period (794-1185) numerous warriors from the Iga and Koga regions sought out instruction from monks to improve their effectiveness during battle. Anyone who was fortunate enough to receive instruction in the monks of Yamabushi or Sohei received instruction on the significance of subterfuge during battle. According to legend, those who first formed Koga groups met around 940. There were originally eight Koga families.

Koga Crest

These were Koga, Ugai, Naikii, Mochizuki, Akutagawa, Ban, Nagano and Ueno. The eight groups were referred to in the "Koga Hachi Tengu" or the "Eight Tengu of Koga." While these families started to expand rapidly during the time, they weren't not thought to be real martial arts (ryu). They were also known by the name of "Gumi," or "Groups," who did not adhere to strict regimens of training and instead learned as they could from any source they could. This was the foundation for a diverse method of training. Eventually the eight original Koga families evolved into 53 separate groups, including, Taro Gumi, Shinpi Gumi, Byaku Gumi, Hiryu Gumi, Sasaki Gumi, Kuruya Gumi, Tatara Gumi, Fukiwara Gumi, Tomo Gumi, Suguwara Gumi, Otomo Gumi, Isshu Gumi, Kawachi Yon Tengu Gumi, Taira Gumi, Kakuryu Gumi and Tachibana Hachi Tengu Gumi.

The SHADOW ARTS FINISH

In the Kamakura period (1185-1333) during which the Ninja arts flourished. The Iga region had its own government, which was overseen by a council. This was beneficial for them since it was known that they were bitter towards external authorities. Koga additionally had a restricted kind of self-government.

Iga Crest

Koga was a part of the Omi region, of which Koga was an area of it was administered by the Rokkaku family. The Rokkaku granted Koga

Koga the power to govern themselves so long as they were in support of the Rokkaku family's efforts. In the end, the power to rule their own affairs gave Iga as well as Koga Ninja the capacity to be independent, hiring them out to anyone they wanted without restrictions. A number of Iga as well as Koga Ninja actually became vassals to clans that were not in their areas, and were able to serve them with aplomb. This meant that various Iga as well as Koga Ninja were frequently competing against each other simply due to their decision to align themselves with rival forces. Although it may appear to be an act of loyalty however, it was not unusual to find the Ninja or the group of Ninja to be devoted to a particular warlord.

The Kamakura time also witnessed the rise of numerous legends and myths about the capabilities and abilities of Ninja. The stories were spawned by the fact that Ninja's actions were not often observed which meant that the enemies of the Ninja could only judge their abilities by the outcomes. Thus, when whole garrisons Samurai suffered from illness or notable people disappeared without trace the blame was placed upon Ninja magic. There was no suspicion of that it was just a case of abduction or poisoning. Instead, the overly religious Japanese people started convincing themselves that the Ninja were possessed of a variety of supernatural powers available to them. They believed that these powers came from connections to the evil "Oni" demons as well as the playful "Tengu" goblins, crows, who were believed to be in alliance with the Ninja because of their ties to the Yamabushi. However, even those who did not believe in Ninja as supernatural entities, those who did not consider Ninja as supernatural beings were not able to underestimate their power as warriors and gathering agents.

Birth of the Shogun

It was during the Kamakura period also produced the first Japan-based Shogun (Military ruler) in Minamoto Yoritomo. In reality, the word "Shogun," which meant "Supreme general" was first utilized to describe military commanders in the first 700 years, when they were fighting tribes that were fighting in northern regions in the nation. However, the word was not used widely for nearly 400 years before Minamoto Yoritomo took over authority over the entire nation in 1185.

Minamoto Yoritomo

Then , in 1192, the Emperor gave him an official title: Shogun. The Shogunate eventually took over the government, assuming all the administrative, judicial and military duties of the nation. The Shogun appointed warlords from the provinces in order to keep complete control. However, the Minamoto replacement, Yoriie, proved unable to achieve the similar. In his time strong members of the Hojo clan was the Regents for the Shogun.

Hojo Crest

First Regent Hojo Tokimasa in a position to control the entire system of Japan's laws as well as its military and revenues as well, which, to all intents and purposes was the only head of Japan. Hojo was the name of the clan. Hojo clan continued to enjoy their status as Regents until the 7th successor Hojo Takatoki who was arrogant and incompetent, tried to imprison the Emperor. The Emperor was able to escape his grasp and began to fight Hojo Takatoki. Hojo leader. At the final battle, Takatoki killed himself on July 4th, 1333. Sadly, despite Takatoki's inept direction the Emperor was not able to restore the imperial rule. In 1338, a new Shogun Ashikaga Takauji took the country's control.

THE WARRING PERIOD

In the Ashikaga Shogunate (1338 1568) The Northern and Southern dynasties engaged in an acrimonious battle against each other. Then, Ninja appeared in full force. They were able to gather information, assassinate important military targets , and relay information to the forces of the alliance.

>

Ashikaga Crest

At this point , the Ninja were accepted as a fact but only for their skillful tactics had won battles. However, despite their role in the wars, once they ended they were not the only ones to be admired. Samurai were awed by the triumph while the Ninja disintegrated into shadows. Also, the period of 15thcentury witnessed the ravages of civil conflict. In 1467, the battle that is known as the Onin war began, which in the majority was fought over what was the successor of the Ashikaga Shogunate, which was ruled by his 7th successor Ashikaga Yoshihisa. The Ashikaga Shogunate was not as powerful as the previous era of governmental rule. The Emperor and his successor, the Shogun his own self had the skills or the power to manage all the feudal dynasties in Japan. The number of ruling families was around 260, which means that in reality, Japan was split up into 260 distinct nations, each of which was ruled by a powerful and independent Daimyo with a huge army. There was no central government they were able to decide how the Daimyo resolved differences with one another during combat.

This was the time of chaos when the Rokkaku clan called for the help by the Koga allies. The Koga came to the aid of the Rokkaku clan together with a small group comprising Iga Ninja. Rokkaku Takayori is the chief of the Rokkaku family, had publicly disobeyed the Shogun Ashikaga Yoshihisa and was forced to flee to the home he had made in Omi province. In the Omi province, the Shogun along with his forces pursuedhim, making camp at Magari village, which is located in the Koga region. Then, the Koga Ninja as well as their Iga allies attacked. The Shogun's army was powerful but they could not withstand the unconventional tactics employed by the Ninja. Shadow warriors struck with fire arrows in dark of the night however they didn't strike at those who were the Shogun's Samurai. They fired their fiery missiles in order to ignite the provisions of the Shogun, hoping to destroy food items water, medical supplies, and other food items.

Ninja fire arrow attack

In the midst of the fire battle an additional group of Ninja came in and dispersed their horses, thereby removing any possibility for a retreat. The Ninja held the army down for several days. Then, as the story unfolded the Shogun was struck with illness when he was in the field and if he didn't have adequate food, water , and medicine, would not survive long. The Shogun's troops tried to escape on foot, but to many Ninja in the forest prevented them from escaping. The Shogun ultimately died, while his troops were decimated. It was a time when the Koga as well as the Iga Ninja were given high praise. The time was referred to as the "Sengoku Jidai,"" or the "Age of the Civil War" (1467 between 1467 and 1603). In the period, Ninja and their special skills were sought after by the. Ninja weren't just used to spy but also in numerous battles led by individual Daimyo in order to control Kyoto. Ninja fire arrows attack 47 It is also in the Muromachi period that Portuguese traders introduced firelocks to Japan (1543). Although guns were a deterrent to the Samurai however, guns were also a source of blessing for the Ninja.

Tokugawa Crest

Utilizing refined black powder and refined black powder, the Ninja could create more durable smoke grenades and explosive land mines, arrows, and hand-held cannons that were small. Ninja were more potent than they had ever been. The legendary general, Tokugawa Ieyasu hired a small number from Koga Ninja to help him get his family members held captive by the clan of Imagawa. The Imagawa held the hostages in order to secure Tokugawa's loyalty to the clan, but after they were released through the Ninja, Tokugawa joined forces with Oda Nobunaga. Nobunaga is frequently referred to as the third unifier of Japan However, his reputation was not one of a nice person. Nobunaga was a formidable military leader who was obsessed by the idea of ruling the entire country. His dream was to bring together Japan under one blade (Tenka Fubu), bringing all the warlords in the country to one with his leadership...whether they like it or not.

NOBUNAGA SEIZES CONTROL

Nobunaga's ambitions for power quickly were realized when, during the Azuchi Momoyama period, he removed his 15th Ashikaga succeeding, Yoshiaki Yoshiaki, out of office and assumed control of the military over Japan and retreated to Kyoto, the capital city. Kyoto. Even though Nobunaga wasn't known as the Shogun however, he was the most powerful person in Japan. A lot of people were unhappy. The Sasaki family employed a massive group consisting of Ninja who came from Iga as well as Koga and then merged along with an entire army composed of Sasaki Samurai. Sasaki's aim was to eliminate Oda Nobunaga. Sasaki divided his army into three separate groups.

Oda Nobunaga

The first group was comprised of Ninja from the families of Mikumo Gumi family, Takanose Gumi Mizuhara Gumi as well as Inui Gumi. The second group was comprised of Koga Ninja from a variety from the families of 53. The third division consisted from Sasaki Samurai. In the fight against Nobunaga the Sasaki's Ninja, Mikumo Iyo No Kami, who was the leader of one of his troops and betrayed Sasaki in order to join Nobunaga. The Sasaki attempt to take on Nobunaga was ultimately unsuccessful.

Nobunaga continued to work to unite the nation. He was a heartless leader, particularly when it was about Buddhists. This was due to the fact that Nobunaga believed on his Christian faith. Then , in 1571, Nobunaga committed the most horrific act. He massacred more than

100,000 men as well as children and women in a frenzied attack on the Buddhist temples located on Mount Hiei and the surrounding region. This was because, from the beginning of Japan's history the warrior-monks from Mount Hiei were heavily involved in the political as well as military activities of the country.

Nobunaga disintegrates the Monastery

In the belief that this was an attack on his authority, Nobunaga destroyed the monastery as well as all the people with connection to the monastery. In the wake of this incident that a number of Ninja were assigned the task of getting rid of this oppressor. One of these Ninja, Sugitani Zenjubo, who was a highly adept warrior of Koga was very close to achieving his goal however, he was not quite close enough. Nobunaga continued to cause havoc across Japan. In the course of his war in the late 1800s, he finally took control of Omi Province, which comprised that region, the Koga region. A Lord from Koga who was known as Takigawa tried to persuade Nobunaga to destroy the Koga families who ruled the province. Takigawa suggested this in hopes that he would be appointed chief of the Omi province once all other family members were wiped out. The Tokugawa Ieyasu supported Nobunaga that this act was not justified. Koga Koga were left in peace ....for the moment.

A few years later, in the Battle of Iga called "Tensho Iga No Ran" (1581) Nobunaga led Katsuyori, his son Katsuyori together with the vast force of Samurai to rid the nation of the savage people and females of Iga. Nobunaga was aware of the effectiveness of combative tactics. He was aware that the Ninja will never accept his rule and thus have to be destroyed. While Katsuyori's Samurai were well-trained however, they could not stand up against the shrewd Ninja who was Iga. In the face of numerous surprise attacks, Katsuyori's army suffered huge losses. After a short time, the battle started the battle ended. Katsuyori and his remaining Samurai fled in shame.

Tensho Iga No Ran

Nobunaga was furious over his son's defeat. He came up with a detailed plan to gather an army. Nobunaga himself headed an army of 4,666 Samurai against the 4000 Ninja who lived in Iga. When he heard about the imminent fight, a lot of Ninja from Koga went to Iga to aid their brothers in the defense of their territories.

Ninja leave their mountain communities to flee

The war lasted just less than an entire week. Even though the warriors from Iga and Koga gave a great fight but they were not able to stand up against the powerful force of Nobunaga. The Ninja ran away in all directions.

People who were able to escape the area sought work among the Lords they worked for during the time. They were accepted as permanently members of these clans from then on. Because of their participation in the war Nobunaga was the one to order the execution of a large number of Koga Ninja and had their villages in Omi destroyed.

Then , in 1582 Oda Nobunaga was murdered by Mitsuhide Akechi who was previously one of Nobunaga's most trusted Samurai and, perhaps, was a Ninja. Though it was regarded as an assassination attempt, Mitsuhide somehow forced Nobunaga to commit seppuku (ritual suicide). It is recorded that Mitsuhide was executed 13 days later in his funeral at the "Incident of Honnoji," but it was reported in whispers from Ninja that he had begun his brand new career as a priest, under"Tenkai. "Tenkai."

Nobunaga is forced to commit Seppuku

Two of Nobunaga's most talented Generals Toyotomi and Tokugawa Ieyasu remained in control however, they were also targeted for assassination. Again, war broke out to decide who would be the next president of the country. Tokugawa was fighting during the time of Nobunaga's death , wanted to go back to his home in Okazaki however, being in danger of his life, He knew he'd require an incredibly strong support. Tokugawa decided to ask to the Ninja commander Hanzo Hattori to be his guardian throughout the duration of his trip. Hanzo was probably the most well-known Ninja known in Japanese history. Hanzo was actually originally a Samurai who transformed into a Ninja.

Hanzo Hattori

A vassal of Tokugawa family, who was educated in all combat techniques and became known as the "Great Lancer" because of his remarkable ability in spear combat.

The first battle Hanzo fought in took place in 1557, at the age of 16 when the Tokugawa Ieyasu fought Uzichijo. His combat skills were amazing. The two most famous fights were in Kanagawa 1570, and Mikatagahara in 1572. Both of these battles were in which he demonstrated that his Ninja abilities were as potent as his combat actions, making him one of the most sought-after Tokugawa shadow warriors. Hattori took the offer and, together with Koga Ninja Taro Shiro , began to gather an army of Iga Ninja as he could locate to become Tokugawa's personal bodyguards. While traveling to Okazaki they had to face many dangers, but in the final, Tokugawa was delivered safely to his home. Ieyasu was rewarded Hanzo with the control over more than 300 rebel Ninja of Iga and Koga and Koga, who all were made permanent vassals of Tokugawa. Hanzo was a loyal servant of the Tokugawa family faithfully up to his passing in 1596, at the death of Fuma Kotaro who was the Ninja pirate.

TOYOTOMI SUSPECTS the power of

The war came to an end in 1590 when Toyotomi Hideyoshi took over the country. While Nobunaga attempted to unite the nation through the use by force, toyotomi concentrated on the intricacies of an organised administration. His nation's structure was composed of warlords from the region who were allowed to remain in their own states in the event that they acted in a peaceful manner with each other. This allowed Toyotomi to pursue his dream. Toyotomi wished to extend the Japanese empire across the entirety of Asia.

Toyotomi Crest

In 1592 and later in 1597 in 1597, he re-entered Korea. He succeeded in taking an extensive portion of territory. Due to his success in the campaigns, Toyotomi started to accumulate wealth that he poured out across the Imperial court, and later to various lords across Japan. He was a hugely popular figure. But, his main goal was to utilize the position he held on the Korean peninsula Korea as a starting point to conquer China. But this dream was not fulfilled. In 1598, Toyotomi's death, he left the title of his estate, land and fortune to his daughter, Hideyori. In the midst of not being mature enough to run the country the country, it was decided Tokugawa would take over until Hideyori reached the age of majority. The problem was that Tokugawa did not intend on transferring power back on the young ruler and instead began to plan to take over the country by himself.

TOKUGAWA SHOGUNATE

In the Battle of Sekigahara (1600) Sekigahara (1600) Ninja returned with a vengeance. Toyotomi Hideyori was finally coming of old age and was able to assume the position of the leader of Japan. Tokugawa was not willing to quit. Again, the warlords of the country were divided into two factions, those who were loyal to the Toyotomi family name and those who remained loyal to Tokugawa. After three years of fights, Tokugawa's troops as well as his secret Ninja forces finally defeated Toyotomi's troops and the Emperor has officially recognized Tokugawa as Shogun for having provided evidence that, although questioned proved that he was being a descendant from Minamoto's family. Minamoto family. But, despite his legendary family lineage, many warlords were committed to restoring his Toyotomi Name to its proper position.

SANADA Uprising

It was the Sanada family of the famous Samurai clan that was exiled from their region for refusing to align with Tokugawa They regrouped in the mountains and secretly plotted to fight Tokugawa. Tokugawa Shogunate. They hid for many years, until they were forced to return in the early hours after one of Tokugawa's Koga Ninja killed the leader of the Sanada family which left the son Sanada Yukimura as clan leader.

Conclusion

After reading this book, you'll have completed a half-century of training to be an ninja of the future. From learning how to build your kiai and being a ninja-like thinker You're now ready for the next stage of your journey.

With all the information you've got right now is the time to find an institution of training that will apply these concepts in practice. It's a bit intimidating at first as there are a myriad of masters and schools in the western and eastern regions of the globe However, you've got the right foundation in place for you to make the commitment to study and grow.

The training you will undergo is long and difficult due to the different levels of ninjutsu mastery are additional specialized levels referred to as belts. The transition from white belt for beginners to the black might not be enough as there are various grades of black belts that are in the higher echelons of Ninjutsu masters.

The highest point of your endeavors, everything must be directed towards becoming acknowledged as an expert. It is the aim of every teacher to help their art and ensure that it is passed on to the next generation. The masters who have been certified are required to make it their life's job to propagate their teachings and discover a student who will continue the practice to the next generation.

We're glad you enjoyed this book!